ENDO

    I have been overweight since I was a kid, and had a hard time losing weight and keeping it off. I had developed type 2 diabetes in my 40s. In my 50s I had become quite ill with all the complications of diabetes: uncontrolled blood sugar, high blood pressure, lots of inflammation, which made it painful to move around. I heard that Wendy Peter was running a focus group for *Encounter Weight Loss*, so I joined. I learned how to eat real food, and making sure I had proper nutrition made me feel so much healthier. I began to understand the issues around food that caused me to emotionally eat, and learning new skills to deal with these issues was something I had never experienced in any other weight loss program before.

    The encouragement to keep on the journey and not look at slip ups as failure made it so much easier to stick with the changes. Weight started coming off, my blood pressure came down, my blood sugar came back to normal, the inflammation in my body started to heal, and the pain went away. Now in my 60s, I feel healthier than I have for years.

Kathy Sanderson

    I was very reluctant about *Encounter Weight Loss* as I was worried that I would fail to lose weight ... again. Yet as I learned about the program and found support through the free online support group, what I discovered was a group of women who would support me and not judge me in my quest to become healthier.

    What I have gained is the support of wonderful women, freedom from cravings, an ability to move more freely, and an increased confidence in myself and my relationship with God. What I have lost is a substantial amount of weight and a feeling of helplessness and hopelessness.

Carol Hill

    I was introduced to *Encounter Weight Loss* in June of 2019. I was highly skeptical as I have tried numerous weight loss programs. I decided

I would take it seriously and change what I was eating. In the past six months I've lost thirty-five pounds. What I have gained is good and godly teaching, the support of others with similar struggles, and strategies to make changes. What I no longer miss is the sugar highs and lows. The cravings for sugar or unhealthy foods. The times of feeling hangry (hungry-angry), particularly in the late afternoon. I appreciate the holistic approach of *Encounter Weight Loss* since food is only part of our wellbeing. It examines our emotions, our relationship to food, what is at the root of issues around food, and most importantly where is God in this relationship. I am thankful for *Encounter Weight Loss* making a difference in my life.

LOIS POPPLESTONE

I have lost 100 pounds since I started the *Encounter Weight Loss* program. I now work for a fitness company helping people transform their lives. I have even been invited onto TV to tell a bit of my story. Thank you for being you and being there in my time of desperation.

BRENDA HOYT BROWN

Wendy is an awesome leader, teacher, and encourager! Overeating can be part of a bigger story. Wendy will help you figure out the bigger story.

JENNIFER LINK OKALUK

Encounter Weight Loss has been instrumental in my healing from emotional eating. This journey with EWL has given me tools and given me a safe space to deal with the pain and trauma that lead me to turn to food for comfort. It's definitely a journey that's life long, but I'm so thankful for this program that has inspired me to find the confident woman that was always inside me. I've lost 55 pounds, but the inward change is worth far more than weight loss.

JENNIFER PETERSON

ENCOUNTER WEIGHT LOSS

WENDY PETER

Encounter Weight Loss by Wendy Peter
Copyright © 2020 by Wendy Peter

Published by Wendy Peter Enterprises
ISBN 978-1-7770-1340-0

All rights reserved. No part of this book may be reproduced or used in any manner without written permission of the copyright owner except for the use of quotations in a book review.

The opinions expressed in this book reflect the personal beliefs of the author and are not intended as medical advice. Please consult your doctor or health care practitioner before starting any weight-loss program.

Bible quotations are from The ESV® Bible (The Holy Bible, English Standard Version®). ESV® Text Edition: 2016. Copyright © 2001 by Crossway, a publishing ministry of Good News Publishers. The ESV® text has been reproduced in cooperation with and by permission of Good News Publishers. Unauthorized reproduction of this publication is prohibited. All rights reserved. The Holy Bible, English Standard Version (ESV) is adapted from the Revised Standard Version of the Bible, copyright Division of Christian Education of the National Council of the Churches of Christ in the U.S.A. All rights reserved.

Cover and interior by Michael P. McIntee

Contact the author at www.encounterweightloss.com or encounterweightloss@icloud.com

1 2 3 4 5 6   25 24 23 22 21 20

This book is dedicated to Susan Conners.

I met Susan when I first started Encounter Weight Loss. She carried a passion for health and fitness and I had hoped to involve her in the development of a fitness program for Encounter Weight Loss as it grew and developed. Susan had a background as a gymnast and had taken sports onto the mission field to serve children in Africa at sport camps.

Tragically, Susan's time on earth was cut short and we did not get to develop a fitness track together. So to honor Susan's memory, part of the proceeds of this book will go to a fund to provide sports equipment for children living in poverty both here and abroad. By purchasing this book, you are helping us to support her cause.

Thank you, Susan, for inspiring me with your example.

CONTENTS

Chapter One	TAKE THE DEEPER JOURNEY	1
Chapter Two	QUICK-FIX OR PERMANENT CHANGE?	9
Chapter Three	E = EAT REAL FOOD	23
Chapter Four	N = NUTRITION MATTERS	39
Chapter Five	C = CONNECT WITH OTHERS	67
Chapter Six	O = OPEN UP	77
Chapter Seven	U = UNDERSTAND YOURSELF	89
Chapter Eight	N = NO GUILT, NO SHAME, NO PERFECTIONISM	123
Chapter Nine	T = TAKE BACK YOUR DREAMS	137
Chapter Ten	E = EXERCISE AS A LIFESTYLE	147
Chapter Eleven	R = RUN TO GOD	161

Acknowledgments ... 177

About the Author ... 179

I am so excited that you have decided to invest in your life with this book.

The teachings and stories in this book were born out of my own journey away from the pain and frustration of the weight-loss industry and the world of quick-fix dieting.

As I got to the root of my own weight-loss puzzle I found myself living from a new place of freedom, courage and self love.

It is my hope that you will find the same freedom and breakthrough for your life as you work though these chapters.

I am delighted to take this journey with you.

—Wendy Peter

•••

www.EncounterWeightLoss.com

Chapter One

TAKE THE DEEPER JOURNEY

Deuteronomy 30:19 This day I call the heavens and the earth as witnesses against you that I have set before you life and death, blessings and curses. Now choose life, so that you and your children may live.

SKINNY OR HEALTHY?

"You are going to be fat... just like your aunties."

The words hung in the air around me, dissolving my innocence about my body, and setting the stage for the years of diet dysfunction that were to come. It was 1976, and I was 11 years old at a family reunion where I had been standing beside my mom as she visited with one of my aunties. The aunty in question had just given my body an appraising glance and made this dire prediction. As I froze in embarrassment, she cemented the words in place with, *"Well, you have the family body type after all."*

"The family body type? I'm going to be fat?"

Up until that moment, I had not given my body a thought. Yet here was a scary prediction planting the first seeds of body shame and self doubt into my identity. I spent the rest of the day looking furtively at my many aunties attending the reunion. Their bodies were larger than some of my teachers' bodies at school, and now I was being informed that not only was that a bad thing, but it was apparently going to happen to me and there was nothing I could do to escape it!

My pursuit of skinny began that day, and like many of you reading this book, I have definitely been around the tree of weight loss many times, and I've been on every diet plan you can imagine. You know the drill. Buy the book, sign up for the program, or get the food list. Psyche yourself up, *"You can do this girl, you know it will be hard, but you have to lose weight."* And so we do… for the first couple of weeks (or the first couple of days, depending upon the severity of the program). Then we give up, because the change was unsustainable, the food disgusting, or the time commitment unrealistic.

And that's how I lived, for years and years, never really happy with my body, turning to emotional eating whenever life became stressful, and not realizing that there were issues under the surface that the weight-loss industry was not addressing.

For instance my desire for "skinny" was far too tied to my self esteem, and no matter how much I wanted to deny it, I had subconsciously attached much of my value and my success to the number on the scale, rather than the state of my health and the content of my character.

Yet the weight-loss industry did not address this issue. In fact for the most part, the industry made it worse, with constant photos of *perfect bodies* set as the standard for us to achieve and unhealthy fad diets promoted as *quick-fixes*.

In addition to this, I grew up in a family that had a generational pattern of alcoholism, where communication was dysfunctional and patterns of stoicism, martyrdom and enabling were passed down just like our family recipes. So by the time I hit adulthood, I had a lot of emotional baggage that I was dragging with me, which often triggered emotional eating. Yet the weight-loss industry was ignoring this major issue that keeps so many in bondage to food, continually promoting diet after diet that only deals with the physical part while ignoring the deeper issues below the surface.

But God in His grace was bringing me answers that have not only transformed my life and my health, but have impacted many others through the Encounter Weight Loss program. These answers came about through a unique set of circumstances that I found myself in which, in the end, led to this book and program.

Over the years, and outside of my issues with my body weight, I had been studying, teaching and writing about emotional healing, or what is called in some circles inner healing. This is a set of principles that help people resolve the issues of their past and step into greater self confidence and freedom.

I had been teaching these principles for quite some time, and had noticed that as I had resolved my own inner issues, the level of emotional and stress eating I was experiencing had diminished dramatically.

Then it all began to come together for me when I began attending weekly weight-loss meetings with a well-known weight-loss company. It wasn't an easy program for me to stick to, as I was always hungry and cranky. But it was the best I had been able to find over the years, so I went regularly.

One day I walked in for the class and I noticed a sign that said, *"New weight-loss class leader needed"*. I thought to myself, "I could do that," as I was already doing a lot of public speaking and had been reasonably successful at their diet. So I applied for the position, and was hired, only to discover that I was being set up by God for something that had been in His heart for the overweight.

You see, the weight-loss company that hired me had a handbook with lessons that corresponded to the calendar year. When I opened the handbook to see the outline of the first lesson I was to teach, I found myself staring at the same words that I had used for the title of chapter one in a book I had recently written on emotional healing. It seemed too odd of a coincidence to ignore, so I decided to weave my own teaching in together with the diet-class outline, to see what would happen.

As I shared my first lesson, it was apparent that the class had never heard anything like what I was teaching. Hope was being released, and the members of the class were being challenged to deal with the issues under the surface instead of only seeing weight loss as just a physical journey. The managers of the company were so impressed by the impact of the material on the class members that they invited me to teach all of my materials on identity, self esteem, and dealing with past baggage. What followed was a season of seeing women who had struggled to lose weight for years now losing significant amounts of weight, because they were now taking the inner journey as well as the outer journey.

We had several women in that class who lost over 100 pounds, and many more lost weight they had never been able to shed. I taught that class for three years, until I began to work full time in a church, and it was time to lay down that commitment.

I did not really expect to teach about weight loss again, but in 2013, God began to stir an idea in my heart with a burden for those who were struggling with obesity, with no help in sight.

As a pastor I could see that their health, and therefore their dreams, were being stolen, and I knew there was a real need for deeper answers than what was being offered by the weight-loss industry.

So in April of 2014, Encounter Weight Loss was born. The theme of the program was Take the Deeper Journey with an invitation for those who were struggling with issues like emotional eating to address what was going on under the surface and to be set free.

For the first two years that I ran the program, we followed a diet that was typical to what you would find in the weight-loss industry. I taught the members to calorie count and eat diet foods in order to lose weight, while also teaching them to deal with underlying issues like emotional eating. For some of my members, that was enough and they were losing weight and keeping it off, while others were still not getting to their goal weight, even if their self esteem was improving.

"The diet itself is too hard."
"I'm always hungry."
"I don't have the self-discipline to do this long term."

These statements were always there among some of the members. I struggled to understand how to help them, because at the time, low-fat eating and calorie counting was still being promoted by the scientific community as the only way to lose weight.

THE MISSING KEY

Ironically, it took a health crisis in my own life to bring about the necessary changes to the Encounter Weight Loss program that have led to long-term success for many of our members. I had been struggling with a chronic pain issue in my hip due to a childhood accident. Over the years, my entire leg had become slightly rotated and was causing unrelenting inflammation and pain. I did not want to take constant pain killers, so I was looking for alternative answers, including specific exercises and diet modifications I could make that might impact my pain levels.

While visiting the local pain clinic, I was informed that if I removed most of the sugar from my diet it might have a positive impact on my nervous system and reduce the chronic pain I was experiencing.

I have always been very skeptical about "food cures" due to my personal history with just about every fad diet that had come out, so I proceeded very cautiously. I began to research the history of sugar consumption and found out that our sugar consumption has increased from 4 pounds per year before the 19th century to over 150 pounds per year. I found out that sugar consumption keeps people on a blood sugar roller coaster of "hungry, tired, and cranky" followed by hyper and stressed.

I discovered that many North Americans are pre-diabetic and that diabetes is spreading through our population like wildfire, even in children. Many scientists are now saying that sugar is the culprit in multiple diseases and auto-immune disorders, and that it was actually sugar, and not fat, that was causing the obesity epidemic in North America. These scientists were now suggesting that the low-fat diet craze of the 1980s had triggered the epidemic, because when the fat was removed from food, the food companies substituted sugar to add flavor and palatability.

To be honest, this was very challenging for me to hear, because it was as if everything I had been taught about weight loss over the years was the opposite of what was beginning to emerge from the scientific community. Eventually, I had studied enough to convince myself to remove most of the sugar from my diet personally, and the results were totally transforming.

I found myself for the first time in my life pursuing healthy instead of skinny. I was no longer feeling deprived all the time. Now I was eating whenever I was hungry, and I could eat until I was gently full. I was eating real, God-made food, and the weight that had always been a struggle not only came off, but it was also now easy to keep it off.

I realized at that point that I would need to bring about a change at Encounter Weight Loss and invited my members to join me in changing our approach. We follow an acronym of core values in the class that spell the word encounter and the first core value had been E=Eat Less Food, thus reflecting the typical diet approach of calorie counting and deprivation. I changed it to **E=Eat Real Food**, and the missing piece of the puzzle fell into place.

Now that everyone was pursuing healthy, rather than skinny, they were operating out of self love and honor for their bodies as a temple, rather than body-shaming, fear and deprivation. They were taking the deeper journey by getting to the root of their emotional eating patterns, developing better relational skills, and learning how to run to God when anxious.

The results have been outstanding. Women who have struggled for 30 and 40 years with their extra weight are now losing it and knowing how to keep it off. Diabetes, high blood pressure and chronic inflammation have healed and emotional eating has been resolved.

One lady from my local class joined with almost 300 pounds to lose. Her dream was to lose enough weight to be able to get into a plane seat and travel on a mission trip to Africa. She had lost almost 200 of those pounds (at the writing of this book), and went to Africa! It's such a joy watching these members step into their dreams.

Now I will say this book is not for everyone. If you only have 10 pounds to lose, and you are looking for six-pack abs and buns of steel, there are many programs out there that may be a better fit for you. Perhaps you only want or need a quick-fix. And while I do take a chapter of the book to focus on exercise as a lifestyle, that is not the primary focus of this book. But if you have struggled on the merry-go-round of dieting, and nothing has really worked for you long term, then this book is for you. It will take you on a deeper journey past the idea of quick-fix and into the realm of permanent change. It will take you beyond the one-dimensional solution offered by the weight-loss industry and into four different encounters that will help you get down to the right motives, build your self-esteem, and bring God into the center of your journey.

At five feet, one inch and approximately 125 pounds, I will never be skinny, but I am healthy! I am slim and comfortable in my own skin. The young girl who set out chasing skinny has now emerged as a woman who knows her true value. I have learned to address emotional eating and its underlying causes in my life, and my relationship with God has taken the place that food used to hold in my heart. So I invite you to join me in experiencing the same kind of transformation from the inside out.

ENCOUNTER WEIGHT LOSS

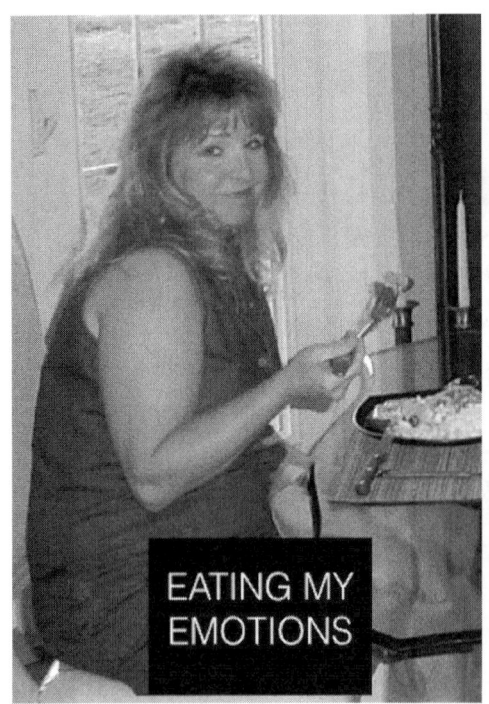

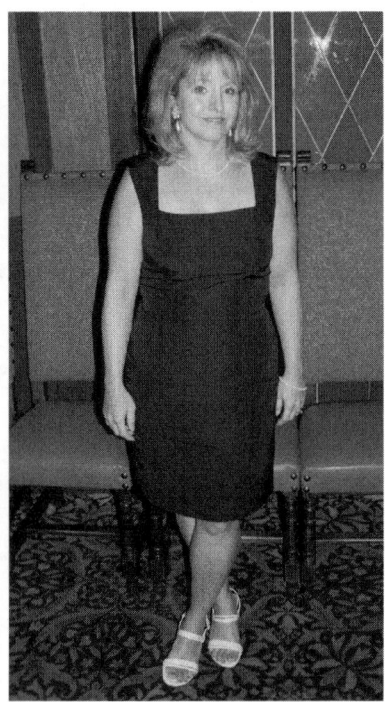

Photos from before and after my weight-loss journey.
Summer 2005.

Chapter Two

QUICK-FIX OR PERMANENT CHANGE?

Proverbs 14:12 There is a way that appears to be right, but in the end it leads to death.

Have you ever heard the statement, "diets don't work"? Most of us have. Yet that doesn't seem to deter us from entering into the madness of following yet another weight-loss fad promising quick results and instant change.

North America's multi-billion dollar weight-loss industry understands this and markets new weight-loss ideas all the time, based on the belief that while nothing prior to their product has really worked for people, (yes, they admit diets don't work) maybe this one will work for you. Companies are even required by law to write the words "Results Not Typical" on the bottom of every before and after photo that they promote, yet it does not deter them in their attempts to pull us into buying their products. It's as if they have secretly agreed to not talk about the elephant in the room called diets don't work, while at the same time presenting us with a new food plan, sales technique or fitness gadget that will draw us into the weight-loss game just one more time.

For the overweight, the frustrated and the tired, this marketing approach is hard to resist. Of course we want hope, of course we are looking for an answer and of course we would love something that would change our situation quickly and painlessly.

However, over time we have become wiser and more cynical, and if you are reading this book, chances are you are looking for something more than what you have experienced in the past. Something that goes deeper than another weight-loss product or fitness gadget. Likely you have tried many diets in the past, without long-term results.

If so, I am happy invite you into a different kind of journey towards weight loss. One that travels through topics that are rarely listed on diet plans or discussed by weight-loss companies and yet are a crucial part of entering into permanent lifestyle change and bringing resolution to core issues. Topics like Understanding Emotional Eating, Identity and Self Esteem, Taking Back Your Dreams, and particularly if you are a person of faith, Taking the Journey with God. These are not topics that are a usual part of weight-loss teaching, yet I fully believe they are a crucial part of a journey towards permanent change.

The journey I am inviting you into will require self honesty and a deeper look inside than perhaps you have taken in the past, yet the payoffs can be life changing. I have heard again and again from the Encounter Weight Loss members that I work with thoughts such as:

"Wow, why didn't anyone ever teach me these things before?"
"No one ever talks about these aspects of weight loss."
"I'm being changed from the inside out."

Much of this change takes place as we come to recognize the ways the weight-loss industry has infiltrated our thinking, and then we move towards realistic, healthier and ultimately more empowering ways of thinking and dealing with food, our bodies and our relationships.

In order to do this, we will need to start with an honest look at the current way we think about weight loss.

Let's begin our journey with the statement "Diets don't work." Is it true, or is it false? Well, actually, many diets do work for a short time, in controlled scientific experiments. The problem is that diets don't work very well for human beings, in terms of us following them in real life, and that is a reality we need to face if we are going to understand and conquer the problem.

We will need to identify the aspects that are not working for us and replace them with an approach that we can be successful with.

Here are the most common things that I hear from clients about why diets do not work for them.

1. Most diets are too hard to stick to
2. Most diets require change that is too extreme
3. Most diets don't work well with our lifestyle
4. Most diets offer no resolution of the emotional triggers for overeating

All of these statements describe what I like to call quick-fix dieting, which is the typical way the weight-loss industry has taught us to think about weight loss. We can understand this problem by looking at the characteristics of a quick-fix diet, and then contrasting those with permanent lifestyle change.

A QUICK-FIX DIET

Starts with the wrong motive

- Weight loss at all costs
- Focus on self and vanity
- Motivation is often pressure from society and others to be thin
- Fear of rejection and feelings of worthlessness as the driving force

Requires extreme sacrifice for a short time

- Rigid rules or prepackaged meals
- Expensive programs you cannot afford long term

- Diet foods you don't like and complicated recipes
- Must be followed blindly; you have no say in the design
- Too much change occurs too quickly, which is hard to sustain

Long-term nutritional / health needs sacrificed

- Requires the use of special supplements, pills, chemically-filled diet foods
- Long-term health implications are ignored
- No connection to long-term quality of life

Social, emotional, spiritual needs ignored

- Isolation from people and normal activities, because diet is so rigid
- God is not part of the process
- No resolve to underlying issues: a surface approach that never deals with the whole picture of why you turn to food for comfort, why certain situations trigger you, and what you need to do to resolve those issues

Not sustainable, too extreme, cost too high

- Only lasts as long as you can keep the external pressure up
- Your body returns to its original condition or worse when you move off the program

Now let's contrast this with:

PERMANENT LIFESTYLE CHANGE

Starts with the right motive

- We tap into long-term health motives (longevity, quality of life)
- Focus is on honoring our body as the temple of God and personal growth
- Self-honor and love are the driving force

QUICK-FIX OR PERMANENT CHANGE

Gradual, moderate effort over long term
- Changes are sustainable because they are gradual
- Room for failure (stumbles are examined for feedback/not judged as failure)
- Affordable program and community that is accessible long term

Long-term nutrition and health needs are invested in
- Knowledge comes through education about nutrition, and personal empowerment comes as understanding of science and nutrition grows
- Overall and individual health needs are respected, and program individualized to reflect this

Social, emotional, spiritual needs honored
- Time is taken to understand underlying issues that trigger overeating
- Trust is built with God and others, and isolation is resolved
- Menu plans are personalized, reflecting likes, dislikes, schedule, and lifestyle
- Identity and self-esteem issues are addressed, moving towards seeing ourselves as God sees us
- New boundaries are set for time management and relationships, balancing one's life, and finding time for God

Transformation is sustainable
- Due to increasing knowledge and individualized adjustments, a powerful new normal has been created, so that core beliefs and motivations are transformed

Before moving on, let's also contrast the language and beliefs of quick-fix dieting with those of permanent lifestyle change. We can see that even the way we talk and think may have been impacted by the weight-loss industry, and the industry can exert an influence on the kind of weight-loss journey we take.

Quick-Fix Language/Beliefs	Permanent Change Language/Beliefs
• I have to	• I choose to
• I can't have that	• I will eat this
• I'm avoiding	• I'm pursuing
• I'm all alone	• I have a community
• Temporary	• Permanent
• Willpower	• God's power
• Rules	• Principles/core values
• I hate my body	• I love myself
• Expensive	• Affordable
• I need the secret	• I need the truth
• Be perfect	• I'm in process
• I'll never get there	• I'm changing every day

Have you noticed something important about the difference between the two columns? The first column reveals a powerless and hopeless mindset, and the second column reveals a powerful and hopeful mindset! This will hopefully be one of your first aha moments while reading this book.

Pause and think about this for a moment. We have been trying to lose weight from a place of feeling powerless and hopeless. It is no wonder that it has not been working for us.

A powerless and hopeless mindset is focused on the external. It functions from blame and a victim mentality, and at its core is driven by fear, and so it manifests as anxiety which drives emotional eating, and thoughts like this:

QUICK-FIX OR PERMANENT CHANGE

"The reason for my problem is out there somewhere and I need to find something out there to fix it."

Whereas a powerful mindset is focused internally, on the power of God and hope as a source for change. At its core it is driven by love and manifests as peace and a steady and courageous pursuit of change from the inside out. A powerful mindset thinks like this:

"The answer to my problem is within, and as I take the time to do this right, I will find the answers and successfully resolve it."

So this book is intended to invite you into a deeper journey that will change the way you think about yourself, your health and your life. This book moves beyond the surface approach of quick-fix dieting, and engages with something much more encompassing— learning how to get healthy, and stay healthy, while honoring the whole person, spirit, soul and body!

Getting off of the diet merry-go-round will free you up to take your time and to explore (with God's help) the weak spots in your relationship with food, yourself, and others. It will allow you the space and grace to uncover the hidden triggers that trip you up again and again in your attempts to lose weight and practice a healthy lifestyle.

While most weight-loss programs are one dimensional and deal only with the physical aspect of calories consumed and burned, the Encounter Weight Loss program takes us into a deeper journey by entering into four different encounters that each reflect an aspect of honoring the whole person, and which work together to create together a deeper, fuller journey into health and freedom.

WHOLE PERSON APPROACH TO WEIGHT LOSS

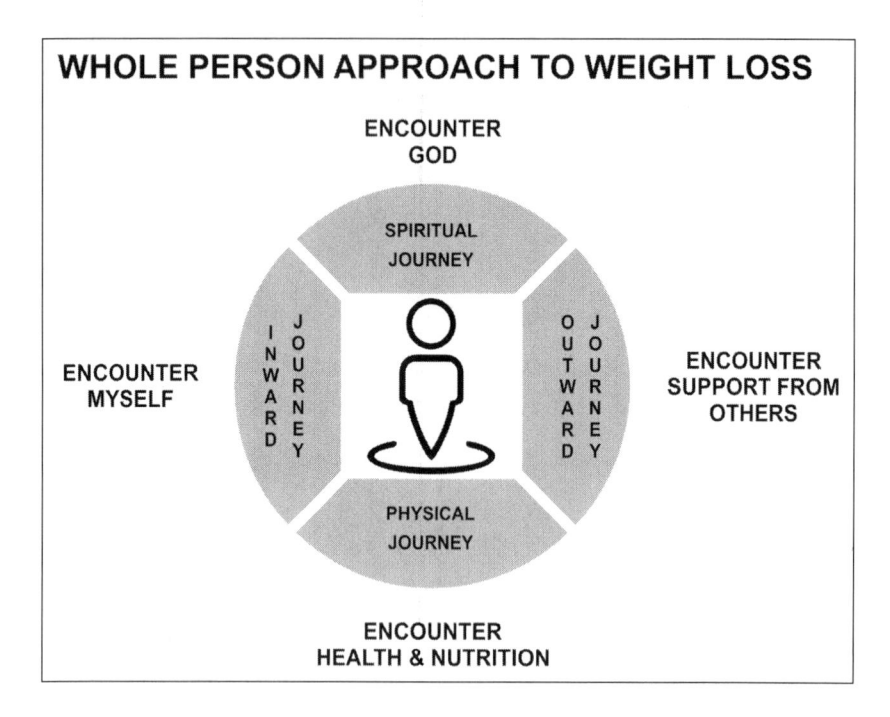

```
                    ENCOUNTER
                       GOD

                  SPIRITUAL
                   JOURNEY

 ENCOUNTER    INWARD    OUTWARD    ENCOUNTER
  MYSELF      JOURNEY   JOURNEY   SUPPORT FROM
                                     OTHERS

                   PHYSICAL
                   JOURNEY

                   ENCOUNTER
               HEALTH & NUTRITION
```

THE FOUR ENCOUNTERS OF ENCOUNTER WEIGHT LOSS

Each of these encounters is a part of the deeper journey that we enter into with Encounter Weight Loss, and each one of these encounters represents an area of your life that can be strengthened and supported to help you gain victory in the area of health and weight loss.

Health and Nutrition Encounter

(The physical journey): we encounter the latest science of health, nutrition, and fitness and we commit ourselves to making new, healthier choices that reflect our increasing knowledge of what is best for us, and which are actually doable within our busy lifestyles.

Encounter with Others

(The outward journey): we encounter community with others (by attending an EWL class in person or online) to gain the support we need, while releasing support to others. We learn to be vulnerable and transparent, sharing our stories, successes and stumbles along the way.

Self Encounter

(The inward journey): we encounter and deal with the root system of emotional eating, including identity issues and the ways we interact with people, stress, disappointment and issues from our past. We examine the relationship recipes that have been passed down in our families that may be tripping us up in our journey towards wholeness.

God Encounter

(The upward journey): we invite God into the process, encountering His love, and learning to surrender to Him. Receiving His grace and empowerment to succeed where we have failed in our own strength in the past. We learn to put food in its place, and run to God when we need comfort.

These four journeys are discussed and applied through a set of core values that spell out the word ENCOUNTER. Throughout the chapters of this book you will be introduced to each of these core values and challenged to make changes in your eating habits, relationships, and identity. As you add each change to the ones before, they will all begin to work together to strengthen your approach to weight loss and help you achieve sustainable transformation.

Let's look at the acronym E.N.C.O.U.N.T.E.R. to give you an overview of where we are headed.

- **E** Eat Real Food
- **N** Nutrition Matters
- **C** Connect With Others
- **O** Open Up
- **U** Understand Yourself
- **N** No Shame, Guilt, Or Perfectionism
- **T** Take Back Your Dreams

E Exercise As A Lifestyle
R Run To God

Some of these values may have been covered in weight-loss books and classes you have engaged with in the past, while others may be entirely new. As mentioned, many of these ideas are completely ignored by the weight-loss industry as a whole. In addition to this, the science of weight loss has changed dramatically in the last three years and may challenge some of the long-held diet rules and beliefs that the media has bombarded you with over the last decades.

However, not only have the old diet rules gone out the window, but so has the white-knuckled calorie counting and deprivation which was the only way we knew how to lose the pounds. So that's good news. The new science of weight loss is helping us lose weight without hunger, and we are seeing a corresponding transformation in our health. In the next two chapters we will explore the core values Eat real food and Nutrition matters and come to understand how this can work for us too.

FROM QUICK-FIX TO PERMANENT CHANGE — MY STORY

I grew up in the 1960s and 1970s with a mom who came from an Irish/English background and who reflected that heritage in our family meals. Meat and potatoes were available for every dinner, with a small portion of canned vegetables on the side. Creamed corn, canned peas, and Harvard beets cut into small squares and coated in a candied sauce. (As kids, we called the Harvard beets poison squares and did whatever we could to dispose of them below the table when mom wasn't looking.)

Salad was hardly ever served and if it was, it contained iceberg lettuce, tomatoes and a can of shrimp on top. (Shrimp? Yes. I have no idea why.) Breakfasts were Corn Flakes or porridge, and lunch was a baloney or ham sandwich on most days. Not the best diet, but certainly not the worst. None of us kids were overweight, because there

QUICK-FIX OR PERMANENT CHANGE

was little added sugar in our food, and we were often told to go outside and play so exercise was a lifestyle.

In fact, if I had not had the negative encounter with my aunty, perhaps I would not have struggled at all. But with my pursuit of skinny, I was the first to buy into the low-fat craze of the 1980s and that's where my trouble began. I still remember buying my first box of Snack-Wells, little chocolate cookies which contained no fat, but were loaded with chemicals and carbohydrates. I never really stopped to think about my health. After all, the products I was buying were called diet foods so they must have been healthy. Or so I thought.

The reality is that our grocery aisles were being flooded with *franken-foods*, man-made chemically-altered concoctions that were quick to make and promised easy weight loss. Insta-noodles, five-minute side dishes, and pre-packaged desserts with low calories. I bought them all, and so did many of my friends.

And we got fat, and then fatter, and then tried to lose it, and it became harder and harder. Our health was also impacted, with extreme PMS symptoms, migraines, rashes, and chronic fatigue becoming normal for many women I knew. Yet a lot of us never really questioned the food. We had a naive trust in the food industry. If the package said it was healthy, it must have been healthy. Sadly it was not!

This was the beginning of my yo-yo dieting years, which eventually led to a place of complete despair and depression as I could not seem to break free from the grip of emotional eating or understand why the harder I tried at dieting, the more overweight I became.

At this point, I would invite you to get a journal that you can write in as we take this journey together through Encounter Weight Loss. I have included activation and journaling questions throughout the book in order for you to get the most out of this journey. If you don't have a journal, grab a piece of paper for today and promise yourself the gift of a fresh, unused journal to record your thoughts as we progress through these core values together.

So let's get started.

ACTIVATION

Let's take a look at whether you have been primarily involved with quick-fix dieting or permanent lifestyle change. Look at the list of quick-fix versus permanent change characteristics below. Circle the quick-fix characteristics that you have bought into in the past.

Starts with the wrong motive

- Weight loss at all costs
- Focus on self and vanity
- Motivation is often pressure from society and others to be thin
- Fear of rejection and feelings of worthlessness as the driving force

Requires extreme sacrifice for a short time

- Rigid rules or prepackaged meals
- Expensive programs you cannot afford long term
- Diet foods you don't like and complicated recipes
- Must be followed blindly; you have no say in the design
- Too much change occurs too quickly, which is hard to sustain

Long-term nutritional / health needs sacrificed

- Requires the use of special supplements, pills, chemically-filled diet foods
- Long-term health implications are ignored
- No connection to long-term quality of life

Social, emotional, spiritual needs ignored

- Isolation from people and normal activities, because diet is so rigid
- God is not part of the process

- No resolve to underlying issues: a surface approach that never deals with the whole picture of why you turn to food for comfort, why certain situations trigger you, and what you need to do to resolve those issues

Not sustainable, too extreme, cost too high
- Only lasts as long as you can keep the external pressure up
- Your body returns to its original condition or worse when you move off the program

Now let's journal

1. What are your thoughts as you look at the approach that you have taken to weight loss in the past?

2. What do you think has been missing from your past attempts at weight loss?

3. I shared two important scenes from my weight-loss journey in this chapter. One was a scene from my childhood and one was a scene from my years trapped in yo-yo dieting. Are there some key scenes that come to mind from your journey with weight loss? Make a brief record of those scenes in your journal.

Chapter Three

E = EAT REAL FOOD

1 Corinthians 6:12 "All things are lawful for me," but not all things are beneficial. "All things are lawful for me," but I will not be enslaved by anything.

In his excellent book *The Seven Pillars of Health*, Dr. Don Colbert says this, "Imagine you have two shelves in your pantry, one that is labeled *"Dead Food"* and the other *"Living Food."* On the *"Dead Food"* shelf is a little tag that reads: *"These foods will make you disease-prone, will cause degenerative diseases such as diabetes, cardiovascular disease, and arthritis, and will make you overweight, fatigued and prone to develop hypertension and high cholesterol."*

But the *"Living Food"* shelf's tag reads: *"these foods will protect your body from cancer, heart disease, all degenerative diseases and obesity, and they will sharpen your mind, energize you and enliven you."*

Which shelf would you choose?

Our grandparents and great grandparents would have no frame of reference for this question. The foods that they ate came from the ground or from the local butcher, and were raised without chemicals, hormones and pesticides, so they never had to make this choice. We on the other hand, have to make this choice every day, whether it's at the grocery store or a restaurant, because in the last 50 years, the food we eat has changed dramatically.

Our ancestors were thinner as a society and enjoyed better overall health than many people do today. Their life expectancy was shorter because they were more likely to die from epidemic, acute and infectious diseases like polio, typhoid, tuberculosis and smallpox, as cures had not yet been found. Yet chronic diseases like diabetes, heart disease, cancer and the myriad of auto-immune diseases we are experiencing today were rarer and obesity was not the norm.

Gary Taubes*, a scientific journalist who has spent the last decade researching the causes of the obesity and chronic disease epidemic in our society, says in his book *The Case Against Sugar*, that diabetes was once a rare disease. He traced its rise through the 1800s and 1900s from just a fraction of one percent of the cases seen at Massachusetts General Hospital to a condition that afflicts nearly one in seven people in the U.S. population (according to the Centers for Disease Control and Prevention.)

In addition a third of all adults are obese, two thirds overweight, and one person in five will die of cancer. The World Health Organization reports that obesity rates have doubled worldwide since 1980. So in spite of our great advances in medicine, these chronic and deadly diseases have been on the rise and have now reached dramatic proportions.

Scientists are taking a whole new look at the underlying causes of these diseases. Where in the past, foods like sugar were seen as a harmless pleasure, scientists are now connecting the dots between the quality of our diets and the staggering increases in these diseases. For instance, says Taubes, sugar consumption has increased from about 4 pounds per year, per person before the 19th century, to a stunning 150+ pounds per year, per person.

According to Taubes and other nutrition researchers, if you were to plot the increase in diabetes and other chronic diseases alongside

E = EAT REAL FOOD

the increase in sugar and processed foods in our diets, there is compelling evidence that these increases run parallel to each other and are showing us an uncomfortable truth.

We are slowly killing ourselves with our toxic, North American diet that is primarily made up of high amounts of sugar. Stop and think about that for a minute. We have added an extra 145 pounds of sugar into our bodies each year. We now eat in two weeks the same amount of sugar that our ancestors ate in one year, so that sugar has now become a large part of our diets.

We have substituted sugar and additives, which contain no nutrition, for the nutrients we formerly consumed as a society, and brought upon ourselves an epidemic of diabetes, heart disease and other serious illnesses. So much for sugar being a harmless pleasure. Nutritionists and scientists are now coming to the conclusion that a calorie is not just a calorie and the type of food we consume has a profound impact on our health and body weight.

We will discuss the scientific mechanics of how that works, and what we can do to reverse it, in our next chapter Nutrition Matters, but for now, let's take a deeper look at the difference between God-made foods, (real foods) and man-made foods (dead foods). In his book *The Seven Pillars of Health*, Dr Colbert went on to contrast the characteristics of Living Foods and Dead Foods.

I have summarized his description for the purposes of this book. Only I will identify them as *Real Foods* versus *Dead Foods*.

REAL FOODS

- Exist in a raw or close-to-raw state.
- Have not been altered in any way. They will mold or rot quickly.
- They are beautifully packaged in wrappers called skins and peels.
- They contain high doses of vitamins, minerals, and phytonutrients. Plants contain more than 100,000 phytonutrients,

minute substances that improve health and cannot be replicated by humans.
- They are recognizable as food.

DEAD FOODS

- They are living foods that have fallen into human hands and been altered in every imaginable way, with additives, chemicals, and bleaches.
- They are intended to last as long as possible at room temperature.
- They are packaged to sell and designed to be addictive.
- They contain large doses of sugar, chemicals, and man-made fats that are created by heating oils until the nutrients die, and then they are reborn as something completely different and often toxic in make-up.
- They are not recognizable as real food.

Sadly, a walk though an average grocery store will reveal that most of the food in the building falls into the category of dead food. An important question that I ask all my members in Encounter Weight Loss is simply this, *"How many steps away from its original state is the food that you put in your grocery cart at the supermarket?"*

How many ingredients does it contain? One? Two? Twenty? God-made foods have one ingredient. For example, an apple contains apple, Cauliflower contains cauliflower. However a Fruit Roll Up that you may innocently buy for your child has a frighteningly long list of ingredients, which include three different versions of sugar within the first four ingredients.

Let's take a look: ingredients in General Mill's Strawberry-Flavored Fruit Roll Ups, in descending order according to amount: Pears from Concentrate, Corn Syrup, Dried Corn Syrup, Sugar, Partially Hydrogenated Cottonseed Oil, Citric Acid, Acetylated Monoglycerides, Fruit Pectin, Dextrose, Malic Acid, Ascorbic Acid, Natural Flavor, Colored Dyes Red #40, Yellows #5 and #6, Blue #1

E = EAT REAL FOOD

Once we see the list right in front of us, it's very disturbing. None of us want to feed our children toxic chemicals. So how did these dead foods creep into our diets? And which ones are the most deadly culprits?

I would recommend a full read of Gary Taubes' book *The Case Against Sugar* for a thorough study of how we have gotten to a point where man-made, processed foods make up such a large part of our diet, but for the purposes of this short chapter I will highlight what I believe are some of the main causes.

Convenience

Our world has become so fast paced in North America and other first-world countries that we feel that we do not have enough time. It seems easier to grab pre-packaged items in the grocery store that are ready to serve, or make a quick stop at a fast-food drive-through restaurant, than it is to purchase fresh produce, cut it up and cook from scratch. At the end of a long day at work, our minds are not on health, they are on trying to juggle our overcommitted lives. Man-made, processed, and pre-packaged foods become the path of least resistance.

Peer pressure and traditions

In many of our families, food means love and sugary desserts and junk food have become part of the traditions we celebrate both in church and family. It can be hard to break these traditions and be the party-pooper who can't enjoy the snacks or the person who doesn't serve them. The peer pressure of these situations can pull us into eating dead, unhealthy foods again and again. Family recipes, cooking styles, and dealing with life using food to celebrate are passed down in families and communities.

Poverty and scarcity of real food

Man-made food and fast food restaurants are not only convenient, they are also cheap food. For a single mom struggling to make ends meet, it can seem beyond reach to purchase God-made, one-ingredient foods. This also impacts the stores in areas where people have lower incomes. It is hard for store owners to spend money bringing in fresh produce, only to have no one buy it, leading to it being thrown out.

I experienced this issue first hand when my husband and I were visiting some friends in a Northern Indigenous community in Canada that was only accessible by plane. Our friends' small children were all suffering from obesity, and I was struggling with a judgmental attitude as I observed their mom giving them sugary juices and pop to drink all day, with no fresh produce in sight.

A deeper look at the situation made me realize that the problem was not as simple as I imagined. It turned out that the local water was undrinkable due to poor sanitation systems and chemical runoff. Then a trip to the only grocery store in the community revealed there was no fresh produce at all for sale. It was too expensive to fly in and spoiled quickly, so it wasn't for sale. A jug of milk was priced at $12 but a bottle of pop was $2. My friends were simply trying to survive in the environment they found themselves in, with very few options available.

Confusion and apathy

Since the 1980s, we have been bombarded with advertising and contrary information about nutrition and health. The expansion of the internet has taken this to extremes. One week, eggs are terrible for us, and the next they are OK. Then we are told fat is killing us, and more recently we are told that some fats are good for us. We have become wearied with the information, worn down and confused. This leaves a feeling of apathy for many, and they no longer look at nutrition labels, or if they do look at them, they are not sure how to interpret the information they find there.

Deceptive advertising

Big food companies exist to make money. They will go to any lengths to do this. They put the word family on high-sugar cereals, use cartoon characters to market those cereals to children, and hide the sugars in the product by using types of sugar with obscure names that do not have to be labeled on the product as actual sugar.

Take for example the Fruit Roll Up that we examined for ingredients. On the nutritional table it states that every 100 grams of Fruit Roll Up contain 38.7 grams of sugar (which is already 9 teaspoons of sugar), but the truth is that there are actually 88 grams or 21 teaspoons of sugar in every 100 grams of Fruit Roll Up, because the other sugar is hidden under the names corn syrup and dried corn syrup. Because of lobbying by the big food companies to control the way food is labeled, packaging can say sugar free on the front of the package and be full of high-fructose corn syrup (which is now hidden in almost every packaged food we consume), and which is beginning to appear, scientists believe, to be the greatest culprit in the current obesity epidemic.

Yet advertisers drown out these realities with lifestyle advertising showing happy, healthy, youthful people drinking something like Coca-Cola, while minimizing the fact that the average size serving (20 ounces) has 16 teaspoons of sugar in it, in the form of high-fructose corn syrup. We would be very unlikely to stir 16 teaspoons of sugar into a glass of water and drink it, but every time we reach for a 20 ounce cola, this is exactly what we are consuming.

To put this into perspective, the World Health Organization has just released new guidelines that state that our sugar consumption should be ideally 5% of our diet and no higher than 10%, which is a recommendation of 4 teaspoons of sugar for women and 9 for men for an entire day. Once we drink even one cola we have exceed that limit by 12 teaspoons of sugar.

High-fructose corn syrup

This product deserves a category of its own as a cause of why we are eating dead foods, because it is so disturbing in its impact on our health. High-fructose corn syrup is a man-made, cheap industrial sugar introduced in the 1970s, originally for sweetening colas.

It has since then crept its way into almost all man-made (dead) foods, and scientists are discovering that it interacts with our liver and our brain differently than other sugars, sending confusing signals to our brain and causing fat storage.

Our North American addiction to soda, candy and processed foods (which are almost all laden with high-fructose corn syrup) has set the stage for excessive overconsumption of this monster-food.

The following is a quote from an article about a Princeton University Study** conducted in 2010: "In the 40 years since the introduction of high-fructose corn syrup as a cost-effective sweetener in the American diet, rates of obesity in the U.S. have skyrocketed, according to the Centers for Disease Control and Prevention. In 1970, around 15 percent of the U.S. population met the definition for obesity; today, roughly one-third of American adults are considered obese, the CDC reported."

High-fructose corn syrup is found in a wide range of foods and beverages including fruit juice, soda, cereal, bread, yogurt, ketchup and mayonnaise. On average, Americans consume 60 pounds of the sweetener per person every year, believed to be the primary culprit in the obesity epidemic.

A 2010 Princeton University research team demonstrated that all sweeteners are not equal when it comes to weight gain: rats with access to high-fructose corn syrup gained significantly more weight than those with access to table sugar, even when their overall caloric intake was the same. In addition to causing significant weight gain in lab animals, long-term consumption of high-fructose corn syrup also led to abnormal increases in body fat, especially in the abdomen, and a rise in circulating blood fats called triglycerides. The researchers say the work sheds light on the factors contributing to obesity trends in the United States:

"Some people have claimed that high-fructose corn syrup is no different than other sweeteners when it comes to weight gain and obesity, but our results make it clear that this just isn't true, at least under the conditions of our tests," said psychology professor Bart Hoebel, who specializes in the neuroscience of appetite, weight and sugar addiction. "When rats are drinking high-fructose corn syrup at levels well below those in soda pop, they're becoming obese — every single one, across the board."

Addiction

Science is showing that high-sugar, processed foods activate the same part of the brain as drugs like cocaine and heroin. In fact, in one study*** rats that were addicted to these drugs were offered a choice of sugar water or the drug and within two days the rats switched over to sugar. There is an addiction cycle driven by these foods. The more of them we eat, the more we crave. Our blood sugar goes on a daily roller coaster ride that drives this addiction cycle, and causes us to become less than rational when our cravings are in full swing.

It is interesting to note that the only nutrient that the Bible clearly warns us against consuming in excess is sugar. This warning is found in Proverbs 25, two times. First in verse 16 *"Have you found honey (sugar), eat only what is sufficient for you, best you vomit it up."* It is apt advice. How many of us have ever binged on sugar and then felt entirely sick afterwards?

And then again at the end of the chapter in verse 27, Solomon warns again *"It is not good to eat too much honey"* and then concludes the chapter with this observation in verse 28: *"He that hath no rule over his own spirit is like a city that is broken down, and without walls."*

I find this biblical connection between sugar and self-control to be accurate as someone who has worked with people for years in the area of weight loss. It has been my observation that those clients of mine who are addicted to sugar, and who try to lose weight while still eating a high-sugar diet, seem to have a very hard time with self control. Yet those who make the lifestyle change of removing sugar and dead, man-made foods from their diet, find that they have recovered their self-control and are no longer feeling as this scripture describes, *"Like a city that is broken down, and without walls."*

I used to think, *"God why did you make us so prone to gaining weight? Why is it so hard to be a normal weight for so many people?"*

He didn't. God made food so that it would work perfectly in our bodies. Rather it is human beings who started making man-made, high-sugar processed foods and created this issue ourselves! Science also bears this out. Our brain will call for and crave more and more food when we live off of junk food and sugar, because our nutritional needs have not been met. I believe that if we would eat only food that God made, obesity would be rare, and the proof of this for me is seeing how many women in my program have been stuck in obesity for years and are now returning to their normal body weight. They are doing it without extreme dieting, but simply by eating primarily God-made foods most of the time.

So let's take a look at that by contrasting the way real foods build your body with the way dead foods impact your body.

What happens when you eat real, living, God-made foods?

- Real foods contain enzymes and fiber that interact properly with your digestive system and allow food to be broken down and move though your body with your digestive system and allow food to be broken down and move through your body with ease.
- Vitamins, antioxidants, minerals and phytonutrients (micro-health protecting agents) are released into your blood stream and build your health, by boosting your immune system and protecting you from disease.
- The leptin in the healthy fats in God made, living foods cause your brain to receive a signal that it is full, and that it is time to stop eating because adequate nutrition has been delivered to your body.

What happens when you eat altered, dead, man-made foods?

- Your body experiences processed, altered and man-made foods like a foreign invader or toxin. Chemicals,

preservatives, food additives, dyes and bleaches enter your blood stream and put pressure on your liver.
- Excessive sugars elevate your insulin levels, causing fat storage signals to be sent. Plaque begins to form in your arteries as your triglycerides remain elevated. Chemicals become stored in your tissues, and your immunity is lowered due to poor nutrition leaving you susceptible to disease.
- Dead/man-made foods send the wrong signals, confusing the brain into thinking that you are full, but because there has been no nutrition delivered to the body, cravings are triggered even though excess calories have been consumed.

Fitness guru and health pioneer Jack LaLane, who lived to be 97 years old, in fantastic health and brimming with energy, when asked what his secret to longevity was answered, "It is very simple. "If God made it, eat it, if man made it, don't."

So, our concluding thought in this chapter is simply this…

If every added ingredient can be seen as a step away from healthy, how many steps away from healthy are the things we are buying each week? How recognizable as food are the items we put in our cart?

EAT REAL FOOD — MY STORY

Nutrition? Building your health on purpose? The truth is, I didn't really understand it or have a clue on how to actually accomplish it for years of my life. I would go through phases where I would buy lots of fresh produce and put it in the fridge, only to see it rot. I ordered bottles of vitamins that would be left on the counter until they were past their expiry date.

Why? Because there was so much confusing information out there, and so much emotional pain in me, and I was hungry, cranky and tired most of the time from low-fat dieting, so that my good intentions barely matched my daily reality. Deep down, I think I identified nutrition with deprivation and punishment and could only think of it in terms of have to rather than want to, and that didn't really change until I changed on the *inside,* and then the outside followed.

I'm telling you all of this, from my personal story, because although the fist few chapters of this book deal with information on healthy eating, it is very hard to sustain the physical journey of healthy eating long term without taking the deeper inward journey and dealing with the underlying issues that drive emotional eating in your life.

So I want you to see it as a starting place, but not an answer unto itself. Most people I have worked with who are overweight know a lot about nutrition, but that doesn't necessarily give them the ability to apply it. We live in an information-driven world, and all you have to do is Google something to get information.

The truth is that we don't need more information, we need an encounter with God's love for us, an encounter with loving ourselves, and an encounter with being loved and supported by others. We need a change in our motive, our identity and our belief system.

People can give you information, but only God can give you a revelation that allows you to apply it successfully to your situation and become a victor, where in the past you felt like a victim.

For me, an important part of my journey is that I had to essentially break off my relationship with sugar as a comfort I turned to whenever I was stressed and unhappy. I'll talk more about that in the chapter on understanding yourself, but for now I just want to remind you that as you read the information in this next core value called N=Nutrition Matters, you may be tempted to simply go back into a quick-fix approach and try to make it into a new set of rules.

I know this because I have watched some of my EWL (Encounter Weight Loss) members do this, and they do lose some weight initially, but because they are only focusing on one part of the program, they eventually get stuck. It's like they are thinking, "new information,

OK, I've got this," while at the same time unconsciously avoiding the other encounters and core values in the program.

And that's OK; we are all human and we tend to start things in our own strength and the ways we are familiar with. The problem with that, however, is if you master the health and nutrition encounter (the information), but never focus on taking the deeper journey and working on all the encounters, you will find yourself after a period of time with many of the old triggers coming back to trip you up and pull you back to where you started.

So my challenge to you is to be gentle with yourself, give yourself time and space to implement the changes, commit firmly to the process and understand that the nutritional piece is only one piece, and it will not sustain your weight loss long term by itself.

That being said, I hope you are excited after reading this chapter and understanding some of the latest science that is showing us that low-fat dieting and deprivation are not the path to permanent weight loss and that it is no longer necessary to be hungry again in order to lose all of your desired weight. You can and will eat foods that are satisfying and be able to watch the pounds fall off. I remember vividly walking around the house saying to myself, "I can't believe I am not hungry, I can't believe I'm losing weight and eating all this real food". And yes, it's true… I did lose my weight that way, and you can too!

ACTIVATION

#1 *What kind of relationship have you had with sugar over the years?*

Has it been a friend, a comforter or a stress reducer? Picture the times you find yourself craving sugar the most. What time of day is it, and what is going on? The answer to this question will give you some clues to your weight loss puzzle as we move forward. (You can add your answers to your journal if you want to keep track of them.)

#2 *Which of the following factors that we identified have played into your weight-loss journey and relationship with unhealthy foods? (Circle those that apply.)*

- Convenience
- Peer pressure and traditions
- Poverty and scarcity of real food
- Confusion and apathy
- Deceptive advertising
- Too many foods with high-fructose corn syrup
- Addiction

#3 *The Seven Day Real-Food Challenge*

Attempt to eat only real (living, God-made) food for the next seven days as best you can. Grocery shop for real food, understanding that every added ingredient takes it another step away from being God made. Start looking at food labels and identify hidden names of sugars that are listed on the label.

I have included a chart with over 50 different names that food companies use for sugar in order to hide it on nutrition labels.

Plan menus with real ingredients, letting go of packagings, sauces, and instant foods, as best you can. If you do need to eat out, choose a restaurant where real food is prepared from scratch.

Cut out all sodas, juices, chocolate milk, junk food or anything else with added sugar. Why juices? Fruit itself is made with built-in fiber, which keeps it from having a negative impact on your blood sugar. With fruit juices, all of the fiber has been removed and it causes an immediate spike in your blood sugar. Drink water, tea and coffee, weaning yourself off diet sodas if possible. Diet sodas can send the wrong signal to the brain, causing cravings and many other problems. They are almost always sweetened with man-made chemicals, although there are a few exceptions. Again, we are not looking here for a quick-fix, so they are not forbidden, but begin to cut back and see how far you can get in seven days.

52 NAMES FOR SUGAR

BLACKSTRAP MOLASSES	BUTTERED SYRUP
CONFECTIONERS SUGAR	CORN SYRUP SOLIDS
DATE SUGAR	DEXTRAN
DIASTIC MALT	ETHYL MALTOL
FLORIDA CRYSTALS	FRUIT JUICE
GALACTOSE	GLUCOSE SOLIDS
GOLDEN SYRUP	HIGH-FRUCTOSE CORN SYRUP
ICING SUGAR	LACTOSE
MALRODEXTRIN	MAPLE SYRUP
MUSCOVADO	PANOCHA
REFINERS'S SYRUP	SORGHUM SYRUP
SUGAR	TURBINADO SUGAR
BARBADOS SUGAR	BEET SUGAR
BROWN SUGAR	CANE JUICE CRYSTALS
CARAMEL	CASTOR SUGAR
CORN SYRUP	DRIED CORN SYRUP
CRYSTALLINE FRUCTOSE	DEMERA SUGAR
DEXTROSE	DIATASE
EVAPORATED CANE JUICE	FRUCTOSE
GLUCOSE	GOLDEN SUGAR
GRAPE SUGAR	HONEY
INVERT SUGAR	MALT SYRUP
MOLASSES	ORGANIC RAW SUGAR
RICE SYRUP	SUCROSE
TREACLE	YELLOW SUGAR
AGAVE NECTAR	BARLEY MALT

Go to your cupboards and fridge and examine some of the foods that are in there. Do you have mostly processed food in your home or real food? Take a look at the labels and ingredient lists. How many grams of carbohydrates are you seeing in your foods? How many ingredients do the foods have? Purge your house of monster foods, with many man-made ingredients, chemicals and additives. Replace artificial sweeteners with natural sweeteners, like Stevia, Truvia, and Swerve.

Make a grocery list in your journal of what you need to buy to enter into the seven day real-food challenge.

If you do not want to wait seven days before moving onto the next step, then simply begin to work on these steps, while also starting the eating plan that you will find at the end of the next chapter.

In the next lesson, N=Nutrition Matters, we will look more deeply into the latest science of weight loss and discover how to reverse the effect that the North American diet has had on our health. We will discover the mechanism within our bodies that causes fat storage and weight gain, and how we can use specific nutritional strategies to reverse that trend, without calorie counting or white-knuckled deprivation.

If you are ready to go onto that lesson today, then you can skip the seven day challenge above, but if you are taking this program one week at a time, I encourage you to take a seven day, real-food challenge that will help you to detox sugar and prepare yourself for an ongoing season of weight loss and restoration of health.

References:

*Gary Taubes, *The Case Against Sugar* (Published by Penguin Random House 2016), Available at Amazon

**Princeton University Princeton University, *A Sweet Problem* (Hilary Parker March 22, 2010. Princeton University News/ Neuro Science Institute)

***British Journal Sports Medicine, *Sugar Addiction: Is It Real? (*British Journal Sports Medicine July 2018)

****Dr Don Colbert, *The Seven Pillars of Health* (Siloam Publishing 2006)

Chapter Four

N = NUTRITION MATTERS

Genesis 1:29 And God said, Behold, I have given you every herb bearing seed, which is upon the face of all the earth, and every tree, in the which is the fruit of a tree yielding seed; to you it shall be for meat.

Genesis 9:3–4 Every moving thing that liveth shall be meat for you; even as the green herb have I given you all things. But flesh with the life thereof, which is the blood thereof, shall ye not eat.

Nutrition matters. In fact it matters so much that it can be a matter of life and death. Most of us would agree with that thought, but we would immediately picture a starving child in Africa with a bloated belly, rather than an overweight North American.

The reality is that obesity is actually a disease of malnutrition or to put it simply under-nutrition, an imbalance of the wrong nutrients in the diet. This *was* well understood by scientists, and successfully treated using this understanding, right up until the Second World War. However, most of the leading nutritional scientists were from Germany. After World War II, much of their expertise was lost, and obesity was newly considered by North American researchers as over-nutrition or eating too much food overall.

This belief also promoted the idea that all calories are created equal, and that you did not need to reduce or adjust any nutrients in your diet, you just needed to eat less food and burn more calories than you ate. For many years this calories in and out model was accepted as the way to lose weight.

This model was based on the law of thermodynamics, which when applied to weight loss, implies that:

- If you burn *more* calories than you consume, you will lose weight.
- If you burn *fewer* calories than you consume, you will gain weight.
- A calorie is a calorie, and all calories will impact your body the same way.

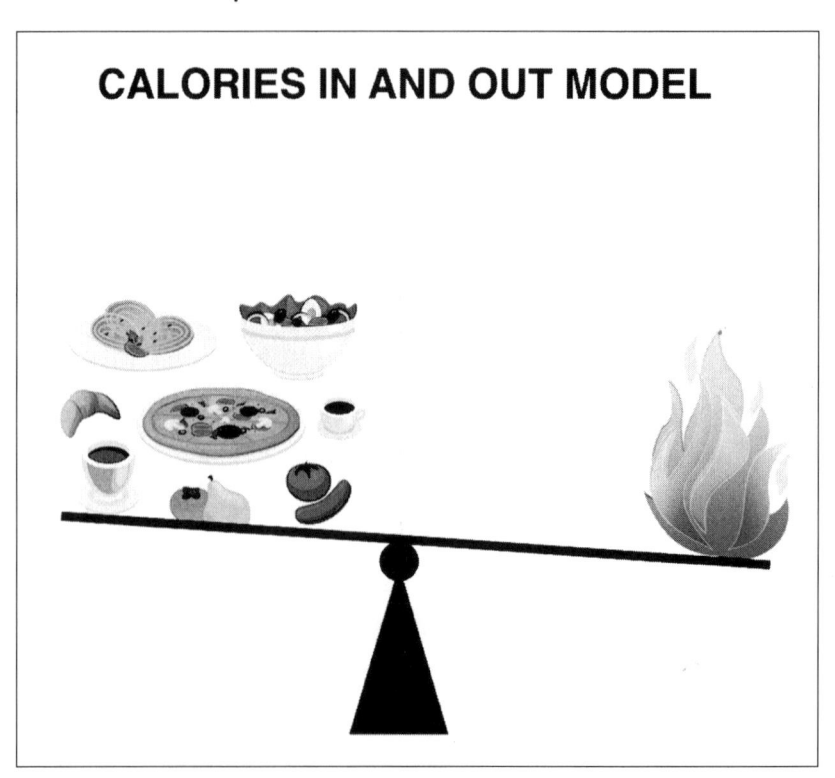

CALORIES IN AND OUT MODEL

N = NUTRITION MATTERS

This teaching, although widely accepted for many years, has had disastrous results. We were told that all calories were created equal, and it did not matter what the percentage of any particular nutrient was in our diet.

Unfortunately, this caused us to gravitate towards a diet high in sugar and refined carbohydrates, because after all, a calorie is a calorie, so just burn it off when you eat it.

Only, it did not work. As we explored in our core value *E=Eat Real Food,* the North American obesity epidemic has developed in response to this imbalance in our diets with millions of people now suffering from malnutrition and unable to lose weight because they continue to believe that all calories are created equal.

The good news is that the old science of weight loss is now being replaced with the recognition that not only is a calorie not just a calorie, but also our bodies respond very differently to various nutrients, by either storing fat or burning fat. The latest nutritional science is saying that the calories in and out model does not work for many people. Most of us already knew this from our own white-knuckled, deprived and frustrating experiences with low-calorie and low-fat dieting. So let's take a look at a simple summary of the latest science.

The Encounter Weight Loss program explores many different aspects of our weight-loss journey of which a part is the science of weight loss. It would take a whole book, and some very complicated terminology, to break down the exact science involved in the mechanism that causes us to store or burn fat. Some of those books have already been written by excellent scientific journalists.

So for the purposes of the Encounter Weight Loss program, I use some basic principles and language to help my members understand the process and get started on their journey towards better health. I then recommend that all members read the books I reference throughout these chapters. I make no apology for this, as the Encounter Weight Loss program encompasses a holistic, whole person approach to weight loss, and the scope of this book needs to encompass that entire message, and not just focus on the science.

I also recognize that one single approach does not work for everyone, and in fact within our program we have members who have tweaked their own weight-loss programs with personalized adjustments such as gluten free, no dairy, intermittent fasting and a few other approaches they have found worked for them.

So what follows below is a summary of what works for most of the people who join our program. It is backed up by good science, and many studies have been done that have confirmed the effectiveness of the science that I reference throughout the book.

At the end of this chapter, I will source some books, websites, and videos that you can use to educate yourself and fine-tune your own journey towards optimum health and weight. In the meantime, the most frequent request I hear from new members is, "tell me what to do, and keep it simple."

NUTRITION BASICS

Our bodies need nutrients in order to grow and function at optimum capacity. There are three basic nutrients contained in the food we consume.

Carbohydrates: are broken down into glucose to give us energy. They also contain fiber and help to remove waste through our bodies. They are found primarily in fruits, vegetables and grains, but also in some nuts, seeds and dairy.

Proteins: build new cells and fix damaged ones in all parts of our bodies. Proteins are necessary for growth. Along with growth and repair, they preserve muscle mass, hormone production, enzyme production, a properly functioning immune system and provide energy if carbohydrates aren't available. Protein is found mostly in meat, eggs, fish, nuts, seeds and beans.

Fats: sustain our health. They are used to build cell membranes and promote absorption of vitamins from the foods we eat. They also make our food taste good. Fats need to be categorized as good or bad, as some promote health and others disease. Good fats include olive oil, coconut oil, avocados, omega 3 oils, and nuts. Trans fats (bad fats) are found in most baked goods and junk food.

When nutrition is balanced within these three nutrients, health is promoted and a normal body weight is maintained. When there is an imbalanced consumption of one of these nutrients, malnutrition and obesity occurs. I know you are not used to seeing the words malnutrition and obesity together, but I want to help you change your thinking and consider the lack of nutrition in a sugar-filled diet, and how that has impacted your health.

In North America we have been eating an imbalanced amount of carbohydrates in the form of sugar and refined flour to the degree that they have become the major part of our diet, with the result being an epidemic of obesity and disease.

As I said in the last chapter, our sugar consumption has gone from 4 pounds per year to over 150 pounds per year per person, so this means that using this measurement alone, our carbohydrate consumption has increased by 3800% since the beginning of the 19th century. This dramatic imbalance of nutrients triggers a fat storage mechanism in our bodies that we need to fully understand if we are to become permanently free from our struggle with weight gain.

UNDERSTANDING THE SWITCH

Nutritional Science researcher Gary Taubes, in his ground breaking book *"Why We Get Fat, And What To Do About It"* states that weight gain is driven very simply by one mechanism in our bodies. A mechanism that we fortunately have control of. This mechanism is related to the way that our bodies *partition* the nutrients we consume to either go into fat storage or be burned as energy.

A naturally thin person's body partitions most of the nutrients they consume to be burned off as energy. This is why they can eat a huge meal and not gain weight, while another person will eat much less and still put on the pounds.

Our bodies naturally partition the nutrients we consume

Naturally heavier person

Her body partitions (sends) the nutrients that she consumes to fat storage

Naturally thin person

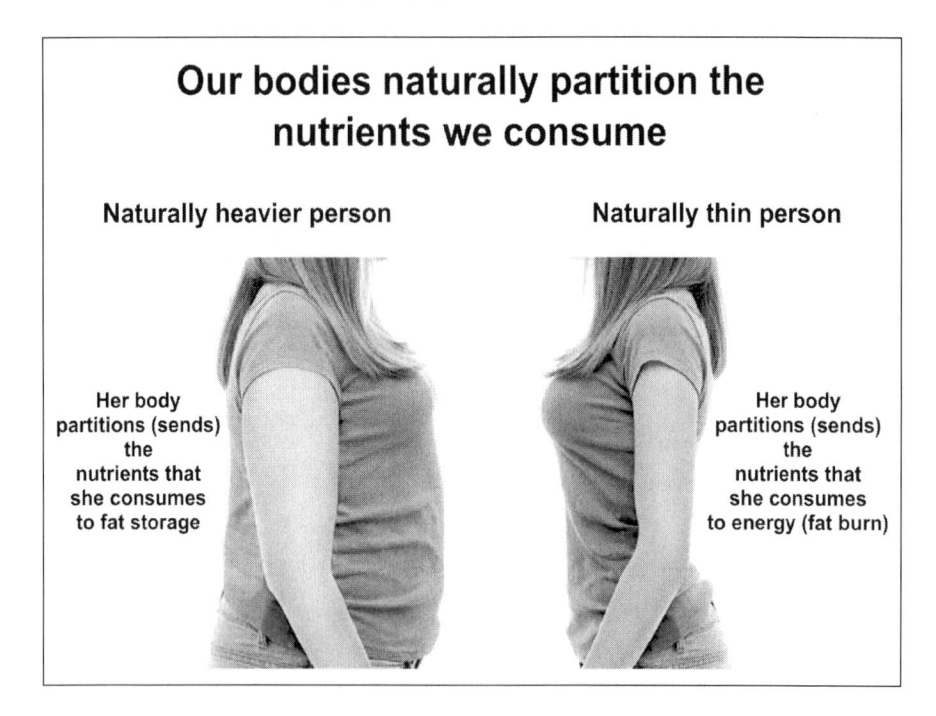

Her body partitions (sends) the nutrients that she consumes to energy (fat burn)

While we cannot change our genetics and the way we naturally partition our nutrients, scientists have discovered that the switch or mechanism that controls this partitioning, either causing fat burn or fat storage, is influenced by the level of insulin in our blood.

Insulin is a hormone produced by the pancreas. What scientists are now discovering is that high insulin levels cause the body to partition nutrients into fat storage and low insulin levels cause the body to partition nutrients into energy to be burned. So in other words, if your insulin is kept low you can be like the person who is naturally thin, who seems to burn everything off, because your body will be partitioning or sending nutrients to be burned as energy.

I simplify this concept for my members at Encounter Weight Loss by saying that high insulin causes our "fat storage door" to be locked, and low insulin levels unlock it and cause our bodies to release stored fat. So this of course begs the questions, "What causes our insulin levels to be high?" and "How can we lower them, so that our fat cells became unlocked and released?"

N = NUTRITION MATTERS

INSULIN LEVELS AND FAT STORAGE

Your body will not burn fat while insulin levels are high

Fat Cells

The answer is fairly simple, and ties in to what we discovered in our last chapter. If we eat more sugar and refined carbohydrates, our body produces more insulin. The typical North American diet is high in sugar and refined carbohydrates. This causes high blood sugar levels and continual fat storage. Thus the obesity epidemic, and our own struggle with weight control.

Sugar and carbohydrate consumption drives up insulin, and insulin drives fat storage!

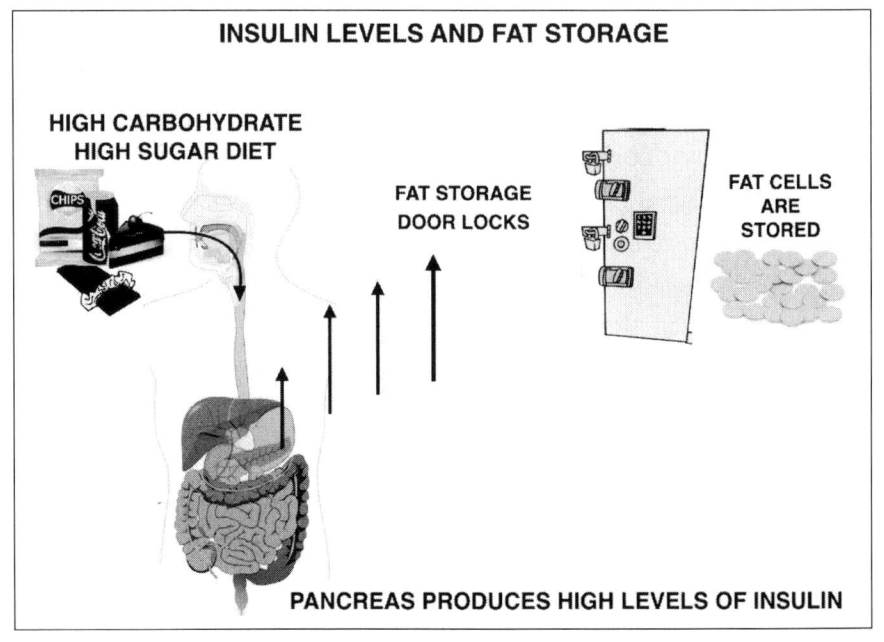

INSULIN LEVELS AND FAT STORAGE

HIGH CARBOHYDRATE
HIGH SUGAR DIET

FAT STORAGE
DOOR LOCKS

FAT CELLS
ARE
STORED

PANCREAS PRODUCES HIGH LEVELS OF INSULIN

In fact, once it hits your blood stream, your body responds exactly the same to carbohydrates as it does to straight sugar.

However, the good news is, that the opposite is also true.

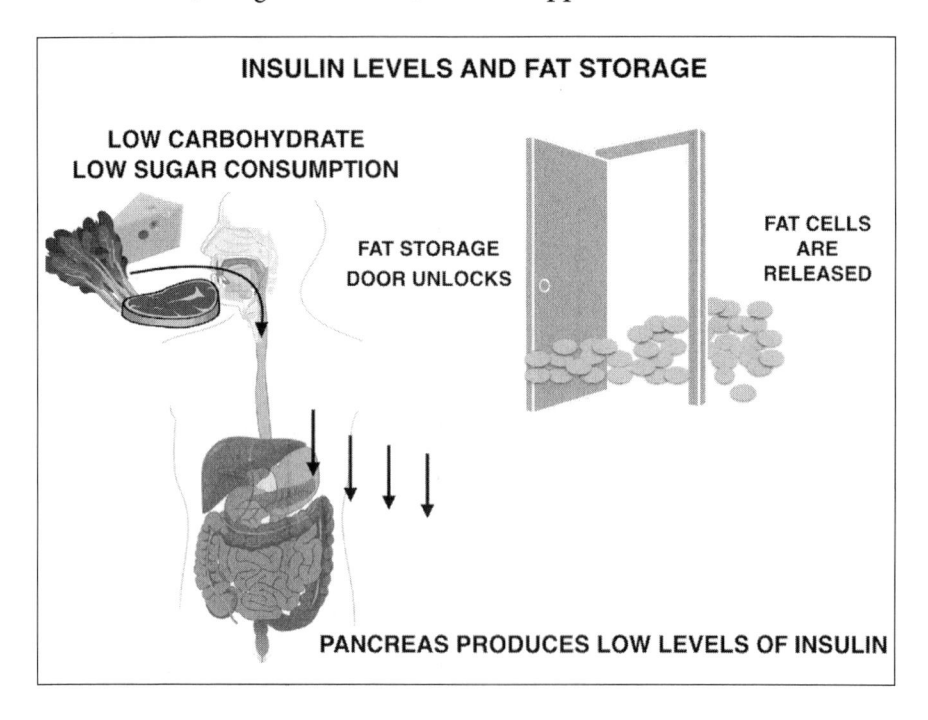

INSULIN LEVELS AND FAT STORAGE

LOW CARBOHYDRATE
LOW SUGAR CONSUMPTION

FAT STORAGE DOOR UNLOCKS

FAT CELLS ARE RELEASED

PANCREAS PRODUCES LOW LEVELS OF INSULIN

Lowering sugar and carbohydrate consumption also lowers your insulin levels and unlocks the "fat storage door."

So, if we were to compare the insulin levels of a person on a typical North American diet with someone on a low sugar, no refined carbohydrates diet over a 24 hour period, we would see that their lower insulin levels would cause their body to metabolize more nutrients into usable energy than into fat storage.

N = NUTRITION MATTERS

Contrast of a 24 hour period on a high carbohydrate diet versus a lower carbohydrate diet.

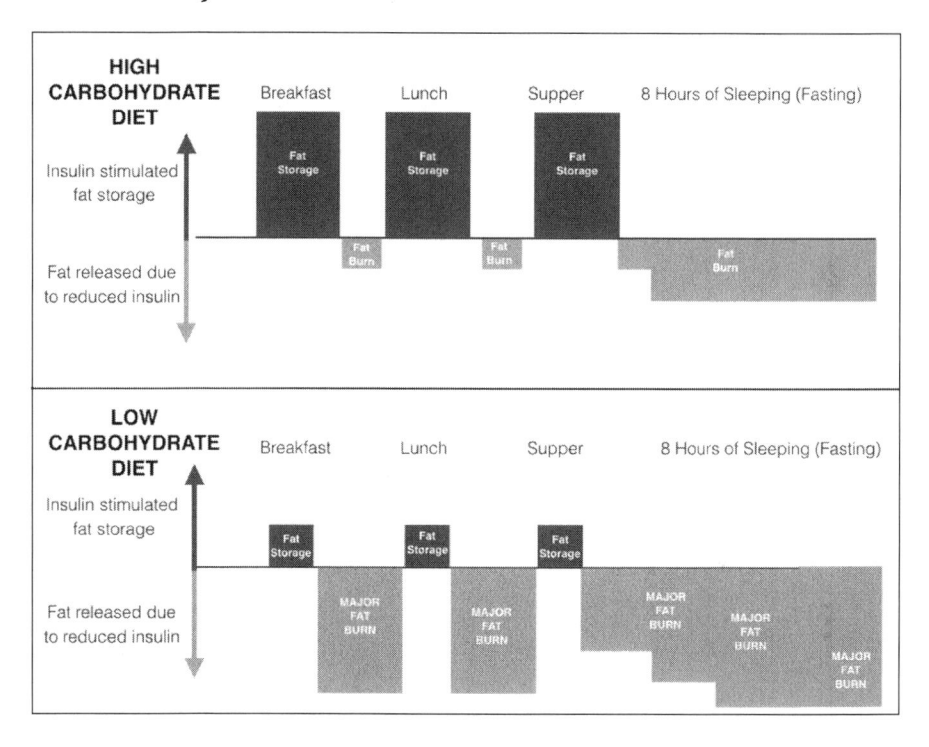

The lower insulin is the switch that makes this happen. In fact the lower the carbohydrate level, the more your body will partition the food you eat into energy, and the more fat your body will burn.

Not only does our body burn more fat when we lower sugar and refined carbohydrates, but we can also be freed from sugar addiction with its insatiable cycle of carbohydrate cravings, mood swings and binge eating.

When we are addicted to sugar, our blood will follow a roller coaster cycle of highs and lows, as our insulin goes way up and then crashes over and over. Not only does this cause fat storage from high insulin, but also every time our blood sugar crashes our body interprets this as an emergency, triggering extreme cravings for more sugar and a loss of self control.

THE SUGAR ADDICTION CYCLE

```
Cravings  ——————→  Eat Carbs/Sugar
   ↑                      ↓
Low Blood            High Blood
  Sugar                 Sugar
   ↑                      ↓
Body Fat            Lots of insulin
Produced   ←—————      released
 Stored
```

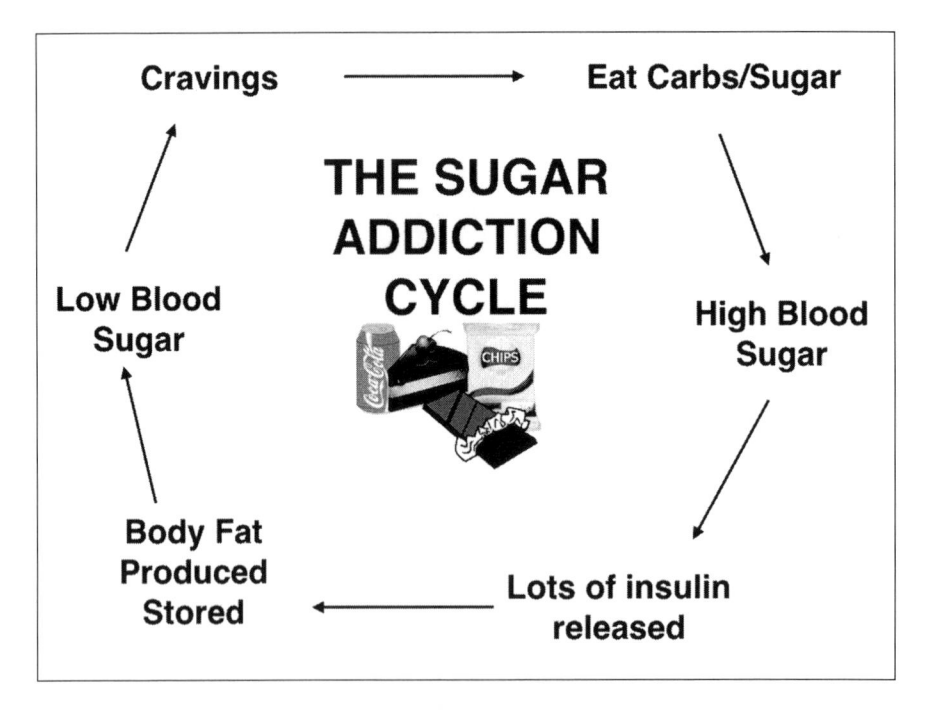

THE SUGAR ADDICTION CYCLE

Once we are free from the highs and lows of this cycle, our mood settles down, our self control returns, and our body begins to release its stored fat.

So now that we are aware of the issue, the next question everyone asks is, "How low should my carbohydrate consumption be"? I wish there were a single answer to that, but with weight loss there is no one size fits all. There are, however, some guidelines I share with members, and then ask them to do what they think will work best for them and adjust accordingly. Then we watch their results together and, using observation and feedback, help them adjust carbohydrate consumption to the right level for their body.

Here are some guidelines to help you get started:

Everyone (including your children) can improve their health by removing added sugars, all obviously refined and processed carbohydrates, and all products containing high-fructose corn syrup.

N = NUTRITION MATTERS

There is some evidence that the single greatest culprit in the obesity epidemic (causing metabolic syndrome and insulin resistance) is high-fructose corn syrup, which has been added to so many foods that we eat.

Some nutritional doctors, including Dr. Robert Lustig in his video *Sugar, the Bitter Truth*, recommend simply removing all high-fructose corn syrup in order to see an improvement in your health. That may or may not be enough of a change for you if you have a lot of weight to lose, but it is certain to help your children and whole family achieve greater nutrition and health.

So the basic place to start is with our first core value: *If God made it, eat it; if man made it, don't."* We also know the World Health Organization has just adjusted its recommendations to reflect that sugar be no more than 5% of our diet. So this means a drastic reduction in the sugar and refined carbohydrates in our diets if we want to lose weight and regain our health.

The following chart is not intended to give medical advice, and simply reflects guidelines I have developed through nutritional study and by working with many members. Everyone has a different threshold of carbohydrate consumption they can tolerate, still lose weight and achieve optimal health.

It is recommended that you do your own research and make adjustments to your diet under the direction of your healthcare professional. At the end of this chapter, I will provide you with a food plan that we follow at Encounter Weight Loss, which will allow you to count your carbohydrates and keep them at a level that will help you first lose weight and then maintain a healthy body weight for the rest of your life.

Take a look at this chart and the explanations that summarize the different levels of carbohydrate intake.

20g	50g	100g	200g	300+ grams
FULL KETOSIS	**MILD KETOSIS**	**STABLE BLOOD SUGAR**		**HIGHER INSULIN LEVELS**
Fast weight loss	Fat as main fuel	Stay thin		Typical American diet
Anti-inflammation	Many health improvements	Maintain healthy body weight		Heart disease, stroke
Pain control	Ongoing weight loss	Good overall health		Diabetes, inflammation
Auto-immune treatment	Improved mood, energy	Wide range of food choices		Depression, low energy
Epilepsy treatment				Metabolic syndrome

HOW LOW SHOULD MY CARBOHYDRATE LEVEL BE?

200-330+ grams of carbohydrates per day:

The typical North American will consume up to 300 grams of carbohydrates per day. This is often consumed in the form of high-fructose corn syrup, sugars, refined carbohydrates (with the fiber taken out), white rice, bread, potatoes, and sodas. All of these foods play havoc with your blood sugar and cause fat storage.

About 100 grams of carbohydrates per day:

Reducing carbohydrates to around 100 grams a day will work for many people with a small amount of weight to lose, or for those who are already thin and want to maintain their weight loss and improve their health.

Make sure that you eat carbohydrates that contain enough fiber, because the fiber can be deducted from the total amount of carbohydrates, to give you a net carbohydrate count. This is because the fiber lowers the impact of the carbohydrates on your blood sugar.

You may need to avoid some fruits, like grapes and bananas, as they are high in sugar and can spike your blood sugar. Normally the

N = NUTRITION MATTERS

fiber in most fruit keeps it from spiking our blood sugar too much, but certain fruits are very high in sugar and you may need to avoid them to keep your carbohydrate level under 100 grams. Experiment and see what works.

If you are not losing weight, lower your carbohydrates, or cut out some of the individual foods you are eating that have a higher dose of carbohydrates in each serving.

You will still likely have some cravings at this level of carbohydrates, but you will also enjoy more freedom of choice in your diet.

If this level works for you in terms of losing weight and keeping it off, then go for it. Interestingly, many members in my class who are at their goal weight, and whom I would overall describe as the healthiest, eat just under 100 grams of carbohydrates per day to maintain their weight loss and still enjoy a varied diet.

It is thought that up until the 19th century, when sugar became widely available, we ate about 70-100 grams of carbohydrates per day. So if you are not insulin resistant and lose weight easily, this may be the right level for you.

50 grams or less of carbohydrates per day:

This level of total carbohydrates will tip your body into a state of fat burn called mild ketosis. Ketosis is a normal metabolic process, something your body does to keep working when it doesn't have enough carbohydrates from food for your cells to burn for energy. It burns fat instead. At this level of carbohydrates, the idea is that your body will burn your fat before it consumes your stored protein, as our bodies are wired this way to protect the muscle mass in our hearts and major systems.

So as part of this process of turning to stored fat as a fuel, your body makes ketones. This means that your body is using mostly fat for fuel as you have given it no choice by lowering your carbohydrates.

Contrary to rumors circulating on the internet, it is not harmful to your body. It is something God built into our systems so that our bodies can switch gears and burn whatever nutrients we have access to. I would like to recommend Doctor Don Colbert's new book *The Keto-Zone* as an educational read that will help you with understanding the science of Ketosis.

Once your body moves into burning ketones, you will lose weight at a slow and steady pace at this level of carbohydrate consumption unless you are insulin resistant.

Numerous websites have sprung up and many cook books have been written that provide fabulous keto recipes that make it easy to eat a lot of different foods and still lose weight.

20 grams or less of carbohydrates per day:

This level of carbohydrate reduction has been used since the 1920s to treat diseases like epilepsy, and more recently studies have shown its effectiveness in improving chronic pain and auto-immune disorders.

Many of our Encounter Weight Loss members start their weight-loss journey by reducing their carbohydrates right down to this level and then adjusting up as they get closer to their goal weight and find their personal threshold of carbohydrates.

This level of carbohydrate consumption will put you into full ketosis, which can be measured using keto-sticks dipped into your urine. (They can be purchased at your pharmacy.) They will turn a bright purple to confirm to you that you are burning primarily fat.

Dr. Colbert recommends everyone start at this level to stay as he calls it being in the keto-zone, and then once you get to your goal weight, slowly increase your carbohydrate amount by five grams per day until you see a weight gain. Then step it back down to your previous level.

This is your personal threshold of carbohydrate tolerance where you will stay healthy and thin. I personally consume between 20-30 grams of carbohydrates per day and that keeps my chronic pain and inflammation from flaring up.

*** If you are suffering from diabetes or other illnesses and are

N = NUTRITION MATTERS

on medication, please have your doctor monitor your progress and choices as medications will often need to be adjusted as you recover.***

*** If you are suffering from a thyroid condition it is not recommended that you lower your carbohydrates below 30-50 grams per day.***

At the end of this chapter, I have included a chart with carbohydrate counts for many foods. You will need to count your carbohydrates if you want to be specific about how many you are consuming.

One way that you can test your level of fat burn is by using ketosticks (mentioned above) which test the level of ketones in your urine. If you are consuming 20 grams of carbohydrate or fewer per day, the sticks will change color from pale pink to purple.

The less sugar/carbohydrates you eat, the darker purple the sticks become. In addition to all of this, I have included a food target diagram at the end of this chapter if you are a visual learner and want to see it laid out in front of you in a way that you can understand. You can download a larger version of this chart in our members-only section of our website along with other key resources if you are part of our online program.

TIPS TO GET YOU STARTED

#1 Check the nutritional information on all of the foods you buy

Don't just look at the sugar count, check the carbohydrates grams on the label as our bodies metabolize carbohydrates just like sugars. If there is fiber in the food, you can deduct it from the total carbohydrate count. This will give you your net carbohydrate count.

Don't be fooled by products labeled

Nutrition Facts

8 servings per container
Serving size   2/3 cup (55g)

Amount per 2/3 cup
Calories   **230**

% DV*	
12%	**Total Fat** 8g
5%	Saturated Fat 1g
	Trans Fat 0g
0%	**Cholesterol** 0mg
7%	**Sodium** 160mg
12%	**Total Carbs** 37g
14%	Dietary Fiber 4g
	Sugars 1g
	Added Sugars 0g
	Protein 3g
10%	Vitamin D 2mcg
20%	Calcium 260mg
45%	Iron 8mg
5%	Potassium 235mg

* Footnote on Daily Values (DV) and calories reference to be inserted here.

low carb or sugar free. Remember what we learned in the last chapter. The food manufacturers will often put a sugar-free label on something when it is full of high-fructose corn syrup. They will hide the sugar grams under another name.

You need to check the nutritional information label

The total carbohydrate count on the nutritional label will always include the sugars even if they are hidden in the ingredient list. You can find many low-carb foods online. I live in Canada and order regularly from a company called Low Carb Canada. They deliver fresh baked low-carb bread right to your door, plus many other products for a very reasonable shipping fee. These products can really help you to stay on track. See www.lowcarbcanada.ca. You can also find low carb products on amazon.com and many other websites. Do a search in your region.

#2 Take the time to prep some foods each week and try out recipes

Hard boiling six eggs, prepping salad ingredients, buying a rotisserie chicken to cut up, and making a basic menu plan for your week can help to keep you on track so that you are ready with a plan in place wherever you are.

Research low-carb/keto recipes on sites like Pinterest. Low-carb recipes such pizza, broccoli cheddar soup, pancakes, and keto fudge will add interest and variety to your diet.

Learning new recipes is part of the lifestyle change you are going to need to make if you are to successfully change your health. I challenge each of my Encounter Weight Loss members to try one new recipe each week. That's 52 new recipes in one year.

#3 Lose your fear of eating fat, and don't overload on protein

After years of hearing low-fat propaganda and advertisements, the idea that fat is good for you can come as a huge shock. I went through a mental battle as I began to follow a high-healthy-fat, low-carb ketogenic diet to treat the chronic pain I was experiencing. The results though spoke for themselves.

After months on the diet, my body had shed its excess fat, and all of my blood tests came out healthier than they had ever been before in my life.

I recommend reading the book *The Big Fat Surprise* by Nina Teicholz, which was released in 2014. She will educate you on the politics behind the low-fat dietary guidelines of the 1980s and the truth about how fat can help and heal your body. I also want to warn you about lowering your fat and carbohydrates at the same time or eating all protein. You might be tempted to think that because low-carb is a good idea, then low-carb and low-fat would be even better. That is not the case.

When you remove the carbohydrates from your diet, you will need to get your nutritional fuel from somewhere else. If you don't get if from carbohydrates, then you must increase your fat intake to compensate. The fats on the food plan at the end of this chapter are healthy fats that are good for you, and they will increase your health. You simply need to move past the low-fat propaganda you have heard for years.

You can help yourself to do that by educating yourself by reading books like the *The Big Fat Surprise*. As for protein, consuming too much protein can cause you to experience diarrhea and keep you from entering into ketosis.

In fact, in one study that Gary Taubes talks about in his book *Why We Get Fat and What To Do About It*, after studying the diet of Inuit people who live on primarily meat, two men followed an all-meat diet for a year and they were in optimal health. This was because the meat had a high fat content. The only time one of them got sick was when he tried eating only lean meat (protein) for a period of time. So educate yourself about fats, and don't be afraid to increase the right ones in your diet. I am on a high-healthy-fat diet to control inflammation, and I am healthier than ever.

#4 Eat enough salt

"What? Raise my salt intake?"

Not exactly, but when you lower your carbohydrate level you end up cutting out a lot of hidden, added salt. So you need to make sure you are keeping your electrolytes in balance. On a low-carb diet, as your insulin levels drop, your body starts shedding excess sodium and water. This is why people will notice a major reduction in bloating once they start to eat fewer carbohydrates.

However, sodium is a very important electrolyte in your body, and you can become ill if your body flushes out too much of it. Side effects of not getting enough salt can include light-headedness, fatigue, constipation and headaches.

#5 Eat your vegetables and some fruits

Non-starchy vegetables should be a daily part of your no-sugar, low-carb diet. Broccoli, cauliflower, spinach, zucchini, bell peppers, and avocados are all rich in nutrients.

In addition to this, many berries are low enough in carbohydrates to include in small amounts, even on a very low-carb program. This core value is called Nutrition Matters and we do not believe in pursuing weight loss at all costs, or weight loss by eating man-made monster foods. So a big part of this program is to improve your overall health through eating highly nutritious food. This means that vegetables and some fruit should be a daily part of your diet.

#6 Don't be obsessive and stressed

High levels of stress can raise the levels of hormones in your body, such as cortisol, which can cause the fat storage door to stay locked. You can find yourself eating the right way, but not losing weight.

The remaining chapters in this book will help you to access key strategies to deal with life. One of the questions I ask all my members is this: *"If you have been an emotional eater, and used food to cope with your emotions and relational issues, how are you going to cope with your emotions and relational issues now that you have given up those foods"*? We must learn a whole new skill set to deal with life, and it is a key part of the Encounter Weight Loss program to learn these skills.

#7 Don't eat too many times per day or too many calories

The reason that lowering your sugar and carbohydrate consumption works so well for weight loss is that your blood sugar is no longer elevated all the time. You can mistakenly override this effect by constantly eating.

Eating nutrient-dense food on a low-carb program should suppress your hunger so that you are not constantly hungry. However, after years of starvation dieting, it can seem too good to be true that you can eat real food, and you can find yourself over doing it.

You shouldn't have to count calories on a low carbohydrate program, but if your weight loss is not moving, then make sure you are waiting long enough between meals, and cut back on portion sizes to feel gently full. Dr. Colbert, in his book *The Keto-Zone*, recommends intermittent fasting as a good strategy to boost your weight loss. An example of this is to stop eating after supper and wait until mid-morning to eat again. This gives your body a long period with low insulin levels and you will burn more fat during this time.

#8 Be careful with artificial sweeteners and sugar alcohols

These products can have negative side effects like diarrhea, constipation, inflammation, and in some cases cause artificial blood sugar spikes. I'll use myself as an example. My body tolerates stevia a natural herb/sweetener very well, also sold as Truvia. I use it in my coffee in the morning, and I also use a baking sweetener called Swerve which contains erythritol, which also has no negative effect on me. However, my body reacts to excess consumption of aspartame with inflammation in all of my joints. Everyone is different, but it is best to avoid man-made sweeteners wherever you can.

One additional warning here. Xylitol is a natural sweetener, but it is toxic to dogs event in tiny amounts and has led to the death of more than one beloved pet. Please be extremely careful about bringing Xylitol into your home if you have pets, or avoid it completely.

#9 Be consistent and patient

Remember Chapter One: The Deeper Journey. I just want to remind you that there is no quick-fix or magic pill that causes instant weigh loss. Although I will say that I have been rather surprised to see that since I started working with members on sugar and carbohydrate reduction rather than low-fat, low calorie plans, I am now hearing women say things like, *"I'm not hungry anymore"* and *"I'm enjoying losing weight."*

After my years in the diet industry working with hungry, cranky, sugar addicted clients, I never thought I would hear those words. But there is more to weight loss than just knowing the science of how to do it.

The truth is that it took us a while to get here, and it will take us some time to get to our goal weight. So I want to end this chapter with a statement that will be a bridge into the rest of our core values and help you move into the deeper journey. It is simply this: "nutrition matters, because you matter." And when you matter to you, nutrition will matter in your life much more than it does now, because we care for, invest in and honor those things we care most about. So hold onto the thought, *"Nutrition matters, because I matter"*, and you will be taking your first steps into the deeper journey.

NUTRITION MATTERS — MY STORY

OK, time for a confession. I don't like vegetables very much. I don't know if I ever will, although I have learned to eat them as part of my diet.

As mentioned in an earlier chapter, I grew up with a few canned vegetables and the occasional salad. So my palette for green leafy vegetables was not developed until much later. I will never forget the first

N = NUTRITION MATTERS

time I purposely made myself a salad to eat in my early twenties. I actually gagged as I tried to eat it. It did not help that it was the 80s and fat was forbidden on the many diets I was trying to follow, so the dressing was not very tasty.

It has been a long journey for me to learn how to make nutrition a part of my permanent lifestyle change. One thing I do is I set a goal to eat salad once a day, another is to eat broccoli a couple of times a week (topped with a cheese sauce) but I have definitely come a long way since my early twenties.

Now in my fifties, I have made a clear connection between the way I fuel my body and my energy level and overall health. As a motivational speaker and coach, this has become increasingly important and not something that I can be casual about, because when I am on the road traveling (which I am very often) it is harder to find fresh low-sugar and healthy food. Even with my best intentions there are times when a family who has invited me for dinner will place a big plate of pasta in front of me.

In order to fulfill the command of Jesus to "eat whatever is set before you" when you travel to represent Him, I usually simply eat it, and it pushes me out of the keto-zone. I then face the challenge of cravings and getting back on track the next day when I eat refined carbohydrates. But I am sharing this with you to say that I understand how challenging it can be. I really do, but I have learned that anything worth having is worth fighting for. Especially my health.

So just like you, I have to navigate the days when I'm tired, the days when I am really busy and take-out food is just easier, and the times when I have to navigate holidays and family events. I do have the occasional time where I don't eat the best, but the Encounter Weight Loss core values have given me the tools to return again and again to the path that will lead to success and a healthy and stable weight.

ACTIVATION

The following food plan is focused on meeting your nutritional needs, while removing sugar and refined carbohydrates. For the most effective weight loss, keep your carbohydrates down to around 20 grams per day. This will give you some momentum as you begin to lose weight. For ongoing weight loss, stay under 50 grams of carbohydrates per day. If you plateau, then lower your carbohydrates back down to around 20 grams per day.

Your diet should be made up from the food list on the following page, plus foods you buy that have a measurable and low-carbohydrate count on them that you can track. Eat when you are hungry, and stop when you are gently full. At the end of this list I have included a chart of carbohydrate counts for common foods. I have also included an Eating on Target diagram that places foods on a target visually in order to help you make healthy choices.

Use this as a grocery shopping list, but then check the chart later in the chapter for the carbohydrate count of each food in order to keep your total daily count where it should be.

GROCERY LIST OF FOODS THAT ARE LOW IN SUGAR AND CARBOHYDRATES

MEAT

- beef (hamburger, steak, roast)
- pork (ham without glaze, bacon)
- lamb, veal
- For processed meats, check the label for carbohydrate count
- poultry (chicken, turkey, duck, other fowl)

FISH AND SHELLFISH

- tuna
- salmon
- catfish

- bass
- trout
- shrimp
- scallops
- crab
- lobster

EGGS

- whole eggs (do not eat egg whites by themselves)

SALADS AND GREENS

- arugula
- bok choy
- cabbage
- chard
- chives
- endive
- greens (collard, mustard, turnip, greens)
- kale
- lettuce
- parsley
- spinach
- radishes

VEGETABLES

- asparagus
- artichokes
- broccoli
- brussels sprouts
- cauliflower
- celery
- cucumber
- eggplant

- beans (green or string)
- leeks
- mushrooms
- okra
- onions
- peppers
- pumpkin
- sprouts
- summer squash
- tomatoes
- wax beans
- zucchini

CHEESE

Carbohydrate count should be less than one gram per serving. Avoid processed cheeses:
- Swiss
- cheddar
- brie
- camembert
- blue
- mozzarella
- cream cheese
- goat cheese
- gruyere

CREAM

Includes heavy cream, 18%, or sour cream.

MAYONNAISE

Use regular mayonnaise or better yet, make your own out of healthy oils. Do not use light mayonnaise.

CONDIMENTS

Use the following condiments and sides sparingly.

Check the labels to make sure they are low in carbohydrates.
- lemon/lime juice
- soy sauce
- pickles (dill)
- vinegar
- mustard

BERRIES

Can be eaten in small amounts.

Use within your carbohydrate allowance. Count the carbohydrates carefully.
- blackberries (5 net carbs per 100 grams)
- strawberries (6 net carbs per 100 grams)
- raspberries (5 net carbs per 100 grams)

FATS AND OILS

Avoid margarine and hydrogenated oils that contain trans fats.
- avocado
- butter
- olive oil
- coconut oil
- coconut butter
- peanut butter
- beef tallow
- chicken fat
- ghee
- non-hydrogenated lard
- macadamia nuts

BEVERAGES

- flavored seltzers with zero carbs
- water, tea or coffee (limit to 3 cups per day or it can interfere with blood sugar)
- diet soda. Some people are affected by diet sodas. They are not forbidden, but they are not encouraged either as they have no nutritional value and can interfere with blood sugar. Use sparingly if at all. Work on switching over to water.

AVOID THE FOLLOWING FOODS COMPLETELY DURING WEIGHT LOSS

Some may be added back in once you increase your carbohydrate threshold when you arrive at your goal weight.

white sugar, brown sugar, honey, maple syrup, molasses, corn syrup, beer, milk, flavored yogurts, fruit juice, sodas, breads, watermelon, pineapple, mangos, bananas, grapes, oranges, peaches, plums, pears, kiwis, cherries, apples, breads, grains, rice, cereals, flour, cornstarch, pastas, muffins, bagels, crackers, pinto beans, lima beans, black beans, carrots, parsnips, peas, potatoes, potato chips, soups, ketchup, relishes

CARBOHYDRATE COUNTS OF MANY FOODS ON OUR PROGRAM

	Grams of CARB.		Grams of CARB.
MEAT		**SEAFOOD**	
Beef (Hamburger, steak, roast)	0	Tuna	0
Pork	0	Salmon	0
Bacon	0.2	Catfish	0
Lamb, Veal	0	Bass	0

N = NUTRITION MATTERS

	Grams of CARB.		Grams of CARB.
POULTRY		Trout	0
Chicken, Turkey, Duck, Fowl	0	Shrimp	0
EGGS		Scallops	0
Whole Eggs	0	Lobster	0
DAIRY/ CREAM			
10%, or 18% (1 TBL)	1		
35% (whip cream, 1 TBL)	0.4		
Sour Cream 1 TBL	0.3		
VEGETABLES (Net carbs, per 1 cup, after deducting fiber)		**VEGETABLES Cont.** (Net carbs, per 1 cup)	
Arugula	0.4	Mushrooms	2.1
Asparagus	2.5	Okra	3.8
Artichokes	9.8	Onions	11
Beans (green or string)	5.9	Parsley	1.8
Bok Choy	0.8	Pumpkin	6.9
Broccoli	3.5	Radishes	2.4
Brussel Sprouts	4.6	Snow Peas	4.9
Cabbage	3.2	Spinach	0.4
Cauliflower	3.0	Sprouts	0.4
Celery	1.9	Sugar Snap Peas	4.9
Chard	0.7	Summer Squash	2.6
Cucumber	3.3	Tomatoes	4
Endive	0	Waxed Beans	4
Eggplant	1.9	Zucchini	2.9
Greens (Collard/mustard/turnip/beet)	0.8		
	5.4	**BERRIES (Per 1 cup)**	
CHEESE (Per 1 ounce serving)	11	Blackberries	6
Brie	0.1	Raspberries	7

	Grams of CARB.		Grams of CARB.
Blue	0.7	Strawberries	8
Camembert	0.1	Blueberries	21
Cheddar	0.4		
Cream Cheese	1.2	**NUTS (Per half cup)**	
Edam cheese	0.5	Macadamia Nuts	3.7
Goat Cheese	1.2	Almonds	6
Gruyere	0.1	Peanuts	5.7
Mozzarella	0.8	Pecans	2.3
Parmesan Cheese	1.2	Walnuts	4
Swiss Cheese	1.5	Cashews	22
FATS and OILS (1 TBL)		**CONDIMENTS 1 TBL**	
Butter	0	Lemon juice	0.7
Olive Oil	0	Soy Sauce	1.2
Coconut Oil	0	Vinegar (Apple, red, white)	0.1
Coconut Butter	0	Vinegar (Balsamic)	2.5
MCT Oil	0	Mustard	0.6
Peanut Butter (no added sugar)	3	Mayonaise	0.1
Beef Tallow	0	Olives (1 medium)	0.2
Ghee (clarified butter)	0	Pickles (1 average)	1
		Avocado (whole)	4

Chapter Five

C = CONNECT WITH OTHERS

Two are better than one; because they have a good reward for their labor. For if they fall, the one will lift up his fellow: but woe to him that is alone when he falleth; for he hath not another to help him up. Ecclesiastes 4:9–11 KJV

We were made for connection. With God, and with each other. So much so, that there is a God-shaped hole in each of us that can only be filled by God Himself. In addition we also have a relational need for companionship, which God summed up in the book of Genesis by saying simply *"It is not good for man to be alone, I will make a helper who is the right fit for him" Genesis 2:18* God said this even though, He as the creator, already had a relationship with Adam. Think about that. God Himself said that man needed connection with someone besides God. God knew that mankind would need relationships with each other in order to thrive.

The breakdown in connection in our first world society has run parallel to the increase in addictions, obesity and other problems in our culture. In spite of the fact that technology has allowed us to contact each other in an instant, emotional disconnection among people is an increasing problem.

There is a decrease in face-to-face connection and real life interaction. Everyone is busy and distracted, even to the point where you will see couples out on a date, gazing at their phones instead of each other. As well, when people do connect online there is often a surface approach to conversations, which can release a sense of envy at the seemingly perfect lives that people seem to portray with special photos, decorating, and super-fit bodies with six-pack abs.

The result of all of this can be a feeling of shame about your less-than-perfect body and your very real life challenges that don't measure up to the success you see online.

It's easy for isolation and loneliness to creep in as our relational need for companionship (which God placed in us) goes unmet. This in turn can be a trigger for overeating in an attempt to find comfort and diminish the feelings of isolation and loneliness that we are experiencing.

In fact, it is interesting to observe that almost all addictive behavior functions in isolation. Think about it in your own life. How often have you binge eaten in front of others? How often in isolation?

Although it may start out in small ways, such as overindulging at a party, it almost always ends in becoming a coping mechanism to comfort negative feelings and deal with stress that we practice in isolation. This is true with many other addictions such as alcohol, drugs, shopping, workaholism or whatever we have turned to. I've even heard it called love hunger.

We know we should go to God and others, but life crowds in and then we grab something to diminish our inner emptiness or calm our stress level. In contrast, when we are not alone, our need for that diminishes greatly. Doctors and psychologists are now identifying isolation and loneliness as root causes in addictive behavior and are recognizing that these ways of coping are often passed down like recipes within families from one generation to another.

So perhaps it will come as no surprise that if I had to choose one core value that is unarguably necessary but often ignored in weight-loss programs it would be this one, Connect With Others.

C = CONNECT WITH OTHERS

Perhaps you have tried to lose weight on your own in the past. How has that worked for you? A recent weight-loss study led by researchers at the University of Illinois discovered that being accountable to others is a critical factor in weight loss success.*

Researcher Catherine J. Metzgar conducted focus groups with 23 women about a year and a half after they completed a weight-loss program to determine which factors helped or hindered dieters' success. While all of the women who participated lost a significant amount of weight on the program, many were unsuccessful at maintaining it after the program ended, Metzgar said. The women who maintained their weight loss were those who indicated that a high level of social support from many sectors was critical in their success.

So let's take a look at why that is, and we'll look at some benefits of connection and strategies for reaching out to find connection with others who want to lose weight.

Connecting with others helps to meet our emotional needs

Most psychologists agree that we have three basic emotional/identity needs:

- Acceptance (a feeling that we belong)
- Significance (a feeling that we have value and purpose)
- Security (a feeling of trust and safety)

When we are connecting in meaningful ways with others and on a regular basis, all three of these inner needs are being met. As we enter into activities such as group discussions, volunteering at our support group, sharing recipes, and exercising together, positive identity messages come back to us that fulfill our emotional needs. Messages like, "I am part of the group", "I have something to contribute", "things will be OK", "people love me, and "I can do this."

We can share our highs, lows, successes and failures with others on the same journey, and as this takes place over time, connection is built. The patterns of isolation that we have been trapped in can be broken, and a powerful new normal established, where we no longer become entrapped by the loneliness and discouragement that have driven our addictive behavior in the past.

Connection with others empowers us spiritually

One of our core values is run to God. His love should be the engine that powers our journey towards permanent health and freedom.

When we pursue God alongside others on the same journey, we are embracing a set of core values together both socially and spiritually. We run to God together, and like a team of joggers running a marathon for a particular cause, we too have a common goal and belief system. Because of this, we can talk about our weight loss in the context of our whole being, including our spirituality.

This is one place that the world has missed in terms of weight loss. People imagine that weight loss is just a physical journey that has nothing to do with the rest of our life. The reality is that you cannot separate the two. The spiritual and the physical are connected, and need to be interconnected in our weight loss journey.

We need to be able to talk about grace, forgiveness, acceptance and even repentance as they would apply to our daily choices. Learning to forgive ourselves for our slip-ups is a part of our spiritual life everywhere else, and it needs to be a part of our weight-loss journey too. When we can use this language in our conversations with others, it brings a sense of spiritual empowerment and wholeness to us as we recognize that all aspects of our lives should intertwine and interconnect rather than being placed in separate boxes.

Connection with others can bring encouragement to us

How much encouragement do you need on a weight-loss journey? You may not realize it, but you may need a lot of personal encouragement, particularly if you have a significant amount of weight to lose.

It is no small task to change an area of our life where we have had

C = CONNECT WITH OTHERS

repeated discouragement. Perhaps we grew up hearing statements like "you will always be overweight" or "you will never change."

These repeated negative messages can become paralyzing over time, until we believe more in our likelihood to fail than we do in our ability to succeed. Being praised for every single pound lost, and every small success along the way, can help us to overcome the negative inner programming that we have carried with us for a long time.

Being part of a group allows us to surround ourselves with people who believe in us, sometimes even more than we believe in ourselves. This can be powerfully motivating, especially during the moments when we stumble or fall.

Connection with others can bring crucial accountability to our journey

How much accountability do you need? This is a key question that needs to be answered if you are going to lose weight and keep it off.

In my work with members over the years, I have come to recognize that almost everyone will have a bad week (or two). However it is not the bad week in itself that knocks people down. It's the irregular attendance and spotty commitment to their group support that knocks people out again and again.

A week of bad choices can set you back a little bit. But like the chutes and ladders game we played as children, more than one week of struggle, on your own without group support, can be the equivalent of landing in a chute that takes you all the way back to the beginning of your weight-loss journey where you gain back your weight and must start over. Whereas the members who come to their weight-loss group week after week have the advantage of a whole team of other members who seemingly reach into the chute and pull them back onto their feet, before they slip too far.

So I believe that connecting with others through weekly weigh-ins, group discussion and support is essential to you making a full lifestyle change.

Of course everyone does not live in my home city in Canada and attend classes here in person, so I started an online Facebook support group for Encounter Weight Loss as an option for those who are far away. This allows you to talk to other members online every day to receive encouragement and coaching when you struggle.

Even if you have no access to the internet where you live, find a partner to take the journey with you. I urge you strongly not to see this core value as *optional,* but to understand that getting a partner or a group to help you cross the finish line is *essential* and may have been the one missing ingredient that has kept you from achieving success. The cost of doing this is only your time, but the payoff is priceless.

CONNECT WITH OTHERS — MY STORY

I had an emotional eating ritual that I started when I was a lonely, angry child. I would buy a bottle of cola, a chocolate bar, and a bag of salt and vinegar chips. It was basically a taste bud party of self-comfort with sweet, salty, crunchy, sour, and fizzy all going on at the same time. I would crawl into the closet by myself and eat the treats while I cried and internalized anything that was bothering me.

It was a ritual that was always practiced in isolation and it set the stage for my later years of emotional eating where I was always alone, always internalizing my emotions and stuffing them down with food.

It got to the point at its worst where food was the first thing I thought about when I woke up in the morning and the last thing I thought about before bed. It was one long, unending meal, and at times it was really out of control. I knew I had a problem, and I honestly thought it was a food problem and that if I could just learn how to like diet food, and eat less, I would lose my weight once and for all.

I had no idea that I did not have a food problem, or even a self-control problem for that matter, rather I had a poor set of skills for dealing with conflict, stress and relationships. A family recipe that was passed

C = CONNECT WITH OTHERS

down of isolation, stuffing emotions, avoiding confrontation and internalizing thoughts and anxieties until the pain was so bad that I medicated myself with food in order to numb the pain.

That recipe was passed down to me by my family alongside the recipe for Yorkshire puddings that my nana made every Sunday to go with the roast beef dinner. The only difference was I made the unhealthy emotional recipe every day, rather than once a week.

I did not find the cure for my unhealthy relational recipe at a weight-loss class, I found it as I launched my first emotional healing class at church.

I found myself in a room of twelve women who all wanted emotional healing, and it was my job to lead them through a book study on the topic. Ironically, I am certain I was among the most emotionally damaged in the room, even though I was asked to be the leader. I did not know the first thing about connecting with others, but now in looking back, I can see that the "book" we studied was the experience of knowing and being known and understood by others, and it began to heal my damaged soul. I had the feeling of no longer being invisible and the message that I was no longer alone in my pain.

So although I did not find help for my emotional eating at a weight-loss group myself, it is my hope that through this book and the Encounter Weight Loss online program, that you *can* find that help as you learn, like I did, to connect with others and break the power of isolation in your life.

ACTIVATION

Tips for establishing a healthy support system

1. Find a partner or group of people who are as committed to change as you are and who hold similar core values.

Resist the temptation to talk or nag someone into this, particularly if that person is your spouse. It's no fun to feel like you are propping up someone else's commitment.

2. Establish the parameters of the commitment you are making, and find out what supports your friend or weight-loss group is offering you.

If you decide to join our online weight-loss program, make sure you commit to posting daily and watching the livestream classes.

If you are isolated from the internet and are doing this with a friend, answer these questions:

- What will we do during our time together? (Weigh-in, trade recipes, go for a walk, study and discuss a core value)
- When will we meet (Be specific about a regular time to meet. This brings a level of long term commitment into play)
- Where will we meet? (Remember that having people over can be a pressure in terms of getting ready and hosting others, so don't put all of the responsibility on yourself. It might be better to meet at a coffee shop or go for a walk together.)
- Why are we doing this? Do we have common goals and beliefs? (It's not a good idea to partner with someone who has a quick-fix, or fad diet mentality if you are pursuing permanent change. If your partner is an atheist and you want to bring God into the journey, it will not be a good fit. Find someone who wants to pursue the ENCOUNTER core values with you.)

3. Decide on the level of accountability you need and want to have.

- Do you need to check in daily? Some of our members post their weigh-ins online, others share food diary pages, others just need to say hello and chat about recipes.
- Do you need someone you can call or reach out to for encouragement if you find yourself really struggling with temptation? Who is this person?

C = CONNECT WITH OTHERS

4. Avoid making promises you cannot keep.

This may sound like a contradiction of my last point, but in actuality it is a reminder to keep things in balance. In our enthusiasm for change, we can mistakenly overcommit to involvement with others by promising things that we are unable to sustain. For example, promising to talk or exercise together every day may or may not be sustainable. Set goals to reach out and connect that have some flexibility built in, rather than make promises that you fail to keep.

5. Try not to prop your partner(s) up.

Sometimes we can find ourselves working harder on someone else's life than they are working on it themselves. While on the one hand we want to encourage and support each other, we also need to allow each other to fail, and find our way back. Doing all of someone's cooking, shopping and supervising their every action is co-dependency rather than support.

6. Know when to move on.

Sometimes we choose the wrong person to partner with and it doesn't work out. Don't be afraid to address this and seek out more support.

References:
* C. J. Metzgar, A. G. Preston, D. L. Miller, S. M. Nickols-Richardson, *Facilitators and Barriers to Weight Loss and Weight Loss Maintenance: a Qualitative Exploration* (September 2014)

Chapter Six

O = OPEN UP

James 5:16 Admit your faults to one another and pray for each other so that you may be healed. The earnest prayer of a righteous man has great power and wonderful results.

We have explored our need for connection with others in our last lesson, and now we will go a little deeper by looking at the core value **Open Up**. For without the ability to open up, we can be physically in a room full of other people and still be utterly alone.

I cannot emphasize enough that far beyond the physical weight-loss information that I have provided in this book, the Encounter Weight Loss core values are the scaffolding that will allow you to go higher and farther than ever before in your quest for a healthy body and freedom from the addiction of food. They are the relational and lifestyle tools that pave the way for your success.

I like to explain it this way: *"Until we learn about, embrace and practice the relational and lifestyle tools expressed in our core values, overeating remains the only tool we use in order to cope."*

So let's talk about opening up, because in case you haven't noticed, many people who are overweight are shut down. They are "closed up". Years of negative experiences and feedback from others have taken their toll. In asking my members who have struggled with a weight problem for years to describe their emotions and experiences while living in our beauty-obsessed culture they use words like rejected, isolated, worthless, shamed, condemned, judged, and invisible, just to name a few.

They often describe feeling trapped in a body that does not reflect who they really are. So you can see how it can become easy to build a wall against those kinds of experiences and feelings and became shut down, closed up and defensive.

Yet the pathway to freedom requires that we reverse this and open up to let God and other people in past the walls we have built so that our God-shaped hole and our people-shaped hole can be filled the way God intended, rather than with food.

This can feel scary, particularly if we have a history of experiencing betrayal and broken trust from others. But just like a baby chick who needs to peck her way out of the egg in order to grow and find freedom, so we too will need to reach out past our protective shell and spread our wings in our quest for freedom. You cannot put something new into something that is sealed shut. When you put a letter into an envelope, it must be open in order to insert the letter. In the same way, if we want to receive the change we are looking for, we need to open ourselves up in several ways. Let's look at some of those ways together:

We need to open up to others

Many of us have become shut down and closed off to others. We have absorbed the pain of rejection, childhood trauma, disappointment, broken trust and many other messages and experiences. When we can find a safe environment to take off our mask and speak honestly from the heart, something transforming begins to happen. The pain that is lodged inside of us begins to spill out.

In fact it can come as a surprise to see how much pain we are carrying. But as we speak honestly and transparently to others, the power of shame and isolation is broken, and our need for connection is met. This in turn leads to a reduction in anxiety and stress, which in turn lowers our addiction to food as a sedative and false sense of comfort.

O = OPEN UP

Telling our story to others also empowers us to reclaim our voice and practice asserting ourselves. The feeling of being invisible and insignificant dissipates as we share our thoughts, ideas, struggles and successes with others. This causes a shift in our identity...

> *"They see me, the real me, and I am important to them. I do not have to cover up or hide who I am. I am free to be me even in my imperfection."*

The lesson in this is that until I show the real me, without my mask on, I will not know what it is to be loved or accepted for my real self. But once I take my mask off and open up to others, my need for acceptance is met as I receive the genuine love and acknowledgment from others that we all long for.

We need to open up to truth

When we have had years of repeated frustration and a lack of success around losing weight, we can become closed off to thinking about the implications of the unhealthy choices we are making. This is known as denial. We may be in denial about how bad our health has become or about the amount of food we are really eating.

The truth is that when you remove sugar from your diet and eat until you are gently full, your body will return to a healthy weight.

If weeks are going by where you are not seeing any weight loss, then it may be that you are in denial about how much you are actually eating, how often you eat, or how much sugar is actually in the food you are consuming.

As I weigh-in people week after week, I have heard many stories about how members *"just can't believe"* that they did not lose weight. Yet once I question them closely, they will often admit to a party here, and a drive-through meal there, and a general disconnect from the plan they started out with.

I have the privilege of watching up front as people work through this with the help of God's love and come through to a greater place of honesty about the choices they are actually making. I believe that we need to open ourselves up to a conversation with God, where He can speak to us about any issue, habit or way we deal with life and people.

When we are open to God in this way, He can lead us *through* and *out* of the patterns that have led us into a dysfunctional relationship with food. This happens as we allow Him to speak to us about anything and everything in our hearts and minds. This may include the way we spend our time, the way we relate to others, what we put in our grocery cart, and when to push away our plate.

Again, I need to emphasize that choosing to turn away from food for comfort goes hand in hand with taking the inner journey where we confront the pain of our past, low self esteem and relationship issues, and this is a process that takes some time. Yet as we continue to walk in truth and open ourselves up to God's correction and direction, I have seen again and again that transformation will come from the inside out.

As assertiveness is traded for people pleasing, exercise is traded for TV watching, and healthy foods are traded for junk food, a healthier, empowered and confident person emerges, one who has a beautiful and intimate, non-defensive relationship with God and others.

We need to be open to a bit of discomfort

As humans, we are creatures of habit and we like to be comfortable. I always use the analogy of a box full of puppies. They like to be warm and comfy. If you take one out of the box, he will cry until you put him back into the warm and comfortable place he was before.

In the same way, getting out of the box of what we are used to can feel uncomfortable. We don't like being uncomfortable, so we try to avoid it. Well, what if I told you that the only way to change is to be uncomfortable?

Think about that for a moment. Discomfort is part of change. If you want to grow a muscle, you go to the gym, and you use that muscle

O = OPEN UP

until it gets really tired. The result is that there are minute little tears throughout the muscle that need to heal. That's why your legs hurt the next day after a work out. As the discomfort heals, the muscle grows and changes and you get stronger.

This principle is the same when it comes to emotional change, social change, or anything new we try. It may feel unfamiliar, uncomfortable, or foreign. It may feel scary to use your voice and confront someone or create a boundary that you need to have in place in order to be successful.

For example, speaking up to a family member or friend and saying, *"No I cannot eat at this fast food restaurant; I need to choose somewhere with healthier choices."*

The discomfort of that moment is the fear that we will be rejected if we assert ourselves. Yet our lack of personal boundaries and our people pleasing may be the very thing that keeps us from successful weight loss. So the only way through to freedom is to embrace the discomfort of changing. Or in the words of one of my good friends Bonita, *"We just need to get comfortable with being uncomfortable for a while."*

Know that discomfort is an indication that change is taking place. We can step into the new, the unknown, and the unfamiliar while knowing we are also stepping into freedom!

We need to be open to trying new foods and experiences

As our horizon begins to expand, we will see that there are many foods that we have never tried. As we try them, we will discover new recipes and ways of cooking. This is an important part of our journey towards success. We need to replace our familiar recipes with new healthier ones. When I removed sugar and processed foods from my diet, I was immediately confronted with my lack of knowledge about how to cook low-carb foods. I realized that my diet had been full of convenience foods, take-out foods, and quick snacks that were full of sugar and trans-fats. This was primarily because I am quite a busy person and I don't have a lot of time to cook. I also do not find cooking relaxing like some of my friends do.

If you are one of those people who love to make complex recipes, you will be excited by all of the possibilities as you create new low-sugar, low-carb recipes in your kitchen. For the rest of us, we can quickly tire of eating low-carb options like eggs over and over, and have a need for more variety in our diet. We will need to enter into a transition of trying out new foods and recipes and adopting the ones that are a good fit with our lifestyle and taste buds.

If you do not make this change, you will be unlikely to succeed long term at permanent lifestyle change. You will still be stuck in a place of quick-fix, trying to eat from just a few choices. I can't say that it was a totally easy or comfortable journey for me, but by the time I was eight months into a low-sugar diet, through trial and error, I had developed a whole new set of recipes that replaced the old family (fattening) standbys.

Lastly, if we are going to step into freedom in the area of weight loss, we will need to be open to one more very important thing.

We need to open up to the love of God

There are two different ways that you can lose weight. One is by law, and the other is by love. A quick-fix mentality is fueled by rules and negative feelings towards yourself. Real transformation comes by a process of coming to love yourself and embrace the love and value that God has for you. There really is a God-shaped hole inside of each of us that only He can fill and He means to fill it with His love.

The love hunger that we have tried to fill with food can only be truly satisfied by God. In addition to this, we need to make the connection between grace and law in the way we view our weight-loss journey. As Christians, we are taught to walk by grace in every area of our lives, yet it seems that when it comes to weight loss people only know how to apply the law, or a list of rules, in their attempts to change. This leads to a cycle of try-hard and give-up dieting and

O = OPEN UP

endless frustration. Yet as the Bible says, it is impossible for mankind to be perfect, and that's the reason that Jesus came to earth and went to the cross for us.

God invites us into a journey of letting Him love us into a place of confidence and wholeness. A place where the fuel for our weight-loss journey is love, honor, and health. All we need to do is make a decision to let Him in, and He will take that journey with us.

We will learn more about this process of opening up to the love of God in our chapter which covers our core value No guilt, shame or perfectionism, but for now I simply want to encourage you to begin to move away from being so hard on yourself and to invite God to release His unconditional love into you.

OPEN UP — MY STORY

Like many of you, my journey with weight loss and the diet industry had brought a lot of shame and frustration into my life. The idea of opening up to others as a pathway to freedom in weight loss never really occurred to me. I understood that attending a weight-loss class on a regular basis could give me a motivational boost, but that is as far as it went.

The concept of talking about my feelings in a group was never presented in any of the diets I had attempted. In fact, if I had not started to lead the emotional healing classes for my church, I may never have made the connection between stuffing my emotions and the binge eating that I practiced whenever I was stressed.

Yet as I learned to share my life story and feelings in that church group, I began to see a shift taking place in my level of self control where food was concerned. It was not easy for me to open up. They say that dysfunctional homes have silent rules such as, *"Don't talk, don't feel, what happens in this house, stays in this house etc."* That unconscious programming had been running me for years, and I had to be intentional about overriding my fear of disclosing myself to others.

As I learned to open myself up to God and others, this brought me into an encounter with truth. The Bible talks about the "spirit of truth" being God's spirit and says in *John 16:13 "But when He, the Spirit of truth, comes, He will guide you into all the truth"*

This encounter with God's spirit, revealed truth to me in two main areas. One area was in my self worth and value. Deep down, even outside of the issues with my body weight, I was suffering from low self esteem. I was bringing more than my physical body to the mirror with me. I was bringing a lot of negative messages and baggage about how I saw myself and allowing those messages to hold me back.

I needed to become open to the love of God for me, and the value He places on me, and the way He sees me. I also needed to be open to facing the truth about the ways I would deceive myself regarding the amount of food I was consuming and its impact on my body weight.

I began to self observe (with God's help), the inner dialogue that would begin in my head, which would lead me to a drive-through take-out meal or a quart of ice cream for self comfort. The spirit of truth was helping me to catch myself in these moments and in a sense confront my own self-destructive behaviors. I learned to take it a step further and open up to others about these self-sabotaging patterns in my life, and for the first time, the cycle of guilt and shame that was driving me in this pattern was arrested.

This process of becoming open to truth eventually led me to study the latest science of weight loss, understand the impact of sugar on our diets and face the fact that I was truly addicted to sugar (and it was destroying my health).

As I continued to study nutrition and encounter truth, I was then ready for the breakthrough that came as a result of being open to experiencing the discomfort of change as the price of lasting transformation. This was necessary to my finally getting different results from those I had experienced for years on the merry-go-round of dieting.

Here are a few discomforts I experienced during that time of breakthrough in my weight-loss journey. You will likely experience many of your own, and I hope that these will give you a few sign posts

O = OPEN UP

along the way to encourage you to simply, in the words of my friend, *be comfortable, with being uncomfortable* for a season.

First of all, I experienced the discomfort of sugar withdrawal as I began to remove it from my diet. I had extreme sugar cravings for a few days, followed by lethargy, brain fog and achy joints. This is often described as the "keto-flu" and is commonly experienced during sugar withdrawal as your body switches off of sugar as a fuel, and detoxes the many food additives and chemicals in the many processed foods you have consumed.

During the first eight months of my switch to a low-sugar/ ketogenic diet, I also experienced many intellectual discomforts. I felt vaguely guilty paying more for some of my favorite new healthy foods. I really had to come into a truth encounter on this one. I had been fine paying top dollar for junk food and take-out food, but now I found myself balking at spending the money for the best foods that would build my health.

I will never forget standing at the cooler at my local store, staring at the eggs, and having to coach myself into buying the free-range eggs that were loaded with healthy fats, but which cost a dollar more than regular eggs.

This was a process I went through with many items. Yet being able to track down and purchase everything from low-sugar ketchup, jam, chocolate, salad dressings, and low-carbohydrate bakery bread has been a key to my success. Without these items at my fingertips, the temptation to turn to sugar would have been much greater. As well, this also played into the self-value message that I sent myself. I needed to value my health, and myself, enough to invest financially in a healthy future.

I also felt uncomfortable taking time to learn new recipes that were not already part of my usual skill set. Having to prop up the recipes and follow detailed instructions left me a little muddled and frustrated at first. Yet those recipes are now the new, healthier versions that I can easily make from memory and can pass down to my children.

Finally, I felt uncomfortable navigating social functions where I had to order my burger with a lettuce wrap instead of a bun, and I was the only one not eating the bread or dessert. I remember vividly the feeling of discomfort and a desire to explain myself to everyone. Yet now it is totally normal for me to order differently from the menu, and I am happily unapologetic about explaining that for health reasons I do not consume white bread and sugar.

I give these few examples so that you can see the progression of change, and how as we open ourselves up to a new choice or experience, we can move through the place of discomfort until the new uncomfortable experience becomes the normal, comfortable routine in our life. This, in a nutshell, is what permanent lifestyle change looks like.

As we close this chapter, I would like to introduce you to a simple meditation that I use in my classes to help members connect with the love of God in a very real way. We use the word *delight* in this meditation because so often we say things like, "Oh, I know, God loves me." Yet, there is still a disconnect. Delight helps us to connect with the intensely positive feelings that God has for us. This meditation will pave the way for some of our future lessons like Understand Yourself and No Guilt, Shame or Perfectionism.

ACTIVATION

Take five minutes each day and practice opening up to God's love by following these three steps in meditative thought and prayer. Some soft instrumental music can help you relax as you open yourself up to His love and a lighted candle can act as a symbol of connection with the light of God's love and truth.

Step #1: *I am*

Take two minutes and meditate on this thought: "I am a spirit. I live in a body and I look out two windows called eyes. I am not my body, and I am not a number on the scale. My value is not in how I look or perform. I am not my past mistakes or failures. I am not my job, my money, or my possessions. I am a spirit, and I am God's child. I release all feelings of failure, fear and regret to Him right now."

Step #2: He delights in me

Take two minutes and meditate on this thought: "God delights in me. He lights up when I walk into the room. His thoughts towards me are not disappointed or angry; His thoughts are wonderful. He accepts me as I am because I am a person in process, both a masterpiece and a work in progress at the same moment. So, He delights in me!" (Simply practice connecting with the idea of God's delight as you rest before Him for a few minutes.)

Step #3: Caught up in His plans

Now, allow your mind to connect with God's promises and possibilities for you. Allow yourself to be caught up in His plans for your future, which include freedom from food addiction, a healthy body, greater mobility, and many other dreams He has for you. Open yourself up to the possibilities and picture yourself stepping into them. What does your amazing new life look like? Picture it in detail.

Finish this meditation with this scripture: *Isaiah 43:19 Behold, I will do a new thing; now it shall spring forth; shall ye not know it? I will even make a way in the wilderness, and rivers in the desert.* See God doing that in your life!

In our next chapter U = Understand Yourself, we will explore how important it is to understand the people, places and things that trigger us and pull us off of our plan. We also will learn how to recognize emotional eating and implement powerful tools and life strategies for dealing with conflict and daily stress, rather than turning to food.

Chapter Seven

U = UNDERSTAND YOURSELF

Psalm 51:6 Behold, you desire truth in the inward parts. You teach me wisdom in the inmost place.

In the years that I have worked with people in the weight-loss industry, I have often heard the statement, "I am an emotional eater", yet it is generally spoken with a vague recognition that there is a problem, and almost no understanding of how to solve it.

This is an area where the weight-loss industry has really dropped the ball. They have not addressed the deeper issues that play into food addiction. If simply knowing how to lose weight scientifically was enough, I would not be writing this book, and there would not be an obesity epidemic in North America and around the world.

So in this chapter, I am going to do my best to help you understand some causes of emotional eating and provide strategies to break free.

As I say to my EWL members whenever we discuss emotional eating, we need to be able to answer the following question, *"If I currently use sweets and junk food to deal with my emotions, then how am I going to deal with my emotions when I give up that food?"*

WHAT IS A TRIGGER EVENT?

Emotional eating can seemingly come out of nowhere. After days, weeks or months of successful choices, a sudden urge to binge eat can surface, leaving us confused, frustrated and vulnerable. This intense desire to turn to food for comfort is often driven by something subconscious coming to the surface. A stressful environment, an unresolved issue, a painful memory, or a negative identity message triggered by an event that pushed that old button.

You may have heard of the "fight or flight" response. Psychologists have observed that whenever we feel attacked or suddenly stressed, we will respond with either flight (wanting to run away) or fight (wanting to defend or attack). They believe this mechanism developed so that ancient mankind could successfully deal with wild animals, but we can find the appearance of the fight or flight response right in the book of Genesis after the fall of man. Let's take a look at that together.

In the book of Genesis, we find Adam and Eve living in a beautiful garden where every need was met and where they had a rich relationship with God and each other. I love the definition of the Hebrew word for peace. Shalom. It translates as "nothing missing, nothing broken." This describes the state that Adam and Eve were living in before the fall. Yet once they ate the forbidden fruit, we immediately see the fight or flight response appear as their deep connection to God was broken.

> *Genesis 3:9 Then the Lord God called to Adam and said to him, "Where are you?" 10 So he said, "I heard Your voice in the garden, and I was afraid because I was naked; and I hid myself." This is the flight mechanism in play: fear, shame and hiding.*

> *Genesis 3: 2 Then the man said, "The woman whom You gave to be with me, she gave me of the tree, and I ate." 13 And the*

U = UNDERSTAND YOURSELF

Lord God said to the woman, "What is this you have done?" The woman said, "The serpent deceived me, and I ate."

This is the fight response in play: defensiveness, blame, and attacking others.

This same fight or flight response can be activated in us, pulling us out of the place of peace by a trigger event. Again, a trigger event is an encounter or event that stirs up something under the surface. It usually has a negative identity message attached to it that is painful and can cause us to feel disconnected from God.

When we are turning to food for comfort (emotional eating), we are trying to dull the pain and make it go away, so we get pulled out of a place of being centered in peace and into either the fight or flight response, both of which trigger emotional eating.

THE FIGHT OR FLIGHT RESPONSE

Fight	*Peace*	*Flight*
Aggression	At rest in my identity	Fear
Blame	Good stress management	Shame
Attack	Feeling connected to God	Isolation
Emotional eating		**Emotional eating**

So, emotional eating is driven by unconscious pressure from within. It comes from issues that are either consciously stressful to us or unresolved within us. I like to use the idea of *layers* of thoughts and beliefs that go deeper and deeper within us to describe the issues involved in emotional eating. Whenever these thoughts and beliefs come to the surface, they can trigger the fight or flight response, and cause emotional eating through our desire to calm the response. The three layers we will talk about here are daily issues, inner attitudes and wounds.

On the surface
"Daily Issues"
- Finances, health, work environment
- Marriage, kids, friends
- Time management, conflicts
- Health, energy levels

Just under the surface
"Inner Attitudes"
- Satisfaction/enjoyment of life
(how things really are)
- Identity
- Spirituality
- Personal growth
- Real status of relationships

Deeper issues below the surface
"Wounds"
- Deep emotional hurts
- Betrayals, losses
- Unfulfilled dreams
- Deep disappointments
- Unactivated purpose
- Unused gifts
- Unconscious deception
regarding my attitudes and actions

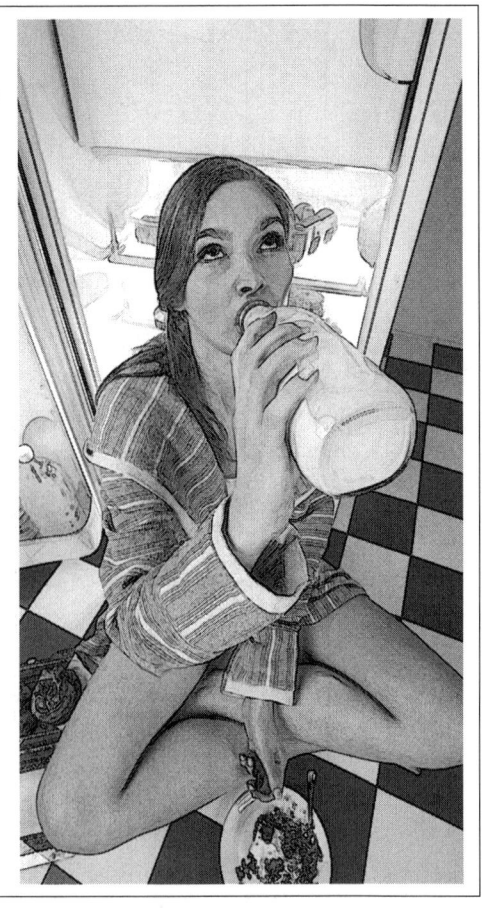

UNDERSTANDING EMOTIONAL EATING

Each of these layers requires a different set of tools and strategies to navigate the stressors, thoughts and beliefs in that layer, without turning to food for comfort. I've illustrated the layers below for you.

So let's take a look at each layer in detail and then identify the strategies needed to conquer emotional eating in that layer. I have divided this chapter into three sections that each deal with one of the layers we have just identified. Each section has detailed strategies and activations for that layer of emotional eating.

Work though each section slowly and thoroughly, incorporating the strategies into your day, answering the deeper questions and

U = UNDERSTAND YOURSELF

setting aside time to work though the activations. This is the longest chapter in the book, and the core of the Encounter Weight Loss message on breaking free from emotional eating. So don't allow this to simply remain as information that you have gathered. I encourage you to read, re-read, underline, and process these ideas. Write in your journal and plan to act on what you find here.

EMOTIONAL EATING
Part #1 The Surface Layer

On the surface layer of life we have our current circumstances. These are the daily issues that we are dealing with right now. These issues can include our finances, relationships, spouse, kids, work, health, and all the things going on around us in the world. Any of these issues can be stressful at any time, and if we do not have good stress-management and lifestyle tools, we can turn to food in order to calm ourselves and manage our stress.

So what are the stress management skills that we need to have in place to deal with this layer? Let's look at three skills that can make a BIG difference in how much stress we are under on a daily basis.

1. Build more margin into your life

What is a margin? A margin is extra space that's created in our lives in order to lower our stress and give us extra time between commitments and the other demands that life brings to us. It's easy to see the margin on this page. It is the space between the written words and the edge of the page. If there was no page margin, the words would be too close to the edge of the page and look crowded.

That's easy to understand, but it's not so easy to find margin in our lives unless we are intentional about creating it. In his excellent book called *Margin: Restoring Emotional, Physical, Financial, and Time Reserves to Overloaded Lives*, Dr. Richard Swenson says: "Margin is the space between our load and our limits. It is the amount allowed beyond that which is needed. It is something held in reserve for contingencies or unanticipated situations. Margin is the gap between rest and exhaustion, the space between breathing freely and suffocating."

There will always be unexpected stressors that come our way, but by creating greater margin in our lives, we can give ourselves more leeway in dealing with stress all around. We can do this by taking back time for ourselves and creating extra time frames around commitments. Below, I have created a list of ways we can carve out more margin for ourselves and thus reduce the stress we are experiencing.

Next to each suggestion, I have asked you to indicate if you are currently doing this, or if you need to create margin in this area. Let's see how much margin you can gain. For instance:

Do you set aside a certain amount of time each morning to simply read, relax, study or pray before you begin your day? This means you don't open up Facebook or look at emails until you take care of this important step.

I currently do this / I need to create this margin

Do you set aside a day of rest or leisure once each week where you do something that gives you joy? If not, you need to in order to take care of your emotional health. Mark this into your calendar as an appointment. Do not let anything push this appointment with yourself off of your calendar. You don't have to justify or defend this appointment to anyone. It is your time to invest in yourself so that you can live a more balanced life.

The Bible calls this day of rest a sabbath and indicates that even God Himself rested. Taking a sabbath day will allow your body, mind and soul to recover from the many demands that have been laid upon you during the week. No sabbath means no time to rest, process or gain perspective. So the practice of taking a day off and being

U = UNDERSTAND YOURSELF

intentional about saying no to anything that feels like a demand is a true gift that you give to your health, both today and in your future.

I currently do this / I need to create this margin

Do you create extra margin around meetings and appointments?
You can do this by planning to arrive 15 minutes early, or by simply marking down your booked appointments as starting 15 minutes before they do. Many times stress comes because we do not factor in the unexpected like a traffic jam or a child who has forgotten something at home. Having those extra minutes of breathing time lowers your stress level dramatically and keeps you free from the anxiety of being rushed, and that plays into overeating. I learned to arrive early for every appointment years ago, and it is now a habit. I always carry a good book with me, and use those extra minutes to read something enjoyable, which also is stress lowering.

I currently do this / I need to create this margin

2. Practice your "No"

I have one friend (Helen) who likes to remind me that, *"No is an answer that does not require an explanation."*

Yet I find that we often have a problem with saying no to people, and this causes all kinds of stress and overcommitment on our part. One strategy that I teach my members is to respond to requests for your time by saying, *"I'll check my calendar and let you know,"* rather than automatically agreeing to every demand placed on you. This allows you to consider whether you have the emotional and physical energy to give to what is being asked. You don't have to explain your calendar to anyone. You can simply say *"I'm sorry, I have looked at my calendar, and I am unable to commit to what you are asking."* You are then able to graciously decline the requests that are too demanding for you.

I currently do this / I need to practice saying no

3. Plan for success

A commonly asked question from our members at Encounter Weight Loss is: how do I navigate social occasions and eating out? And the answer to this question comes from an old adage that is often spoken around weight loss circles. *"If you fail to plan, you plan to fail"*.

Planning means that you created enough margin in your life to focus on and fulfill the tasks needed to ensure success on your weight loss program.

Social occasions are full of emotional triggers and identity messages and questions such as, "Am I accepted? Am I significant? Do people like me?" All of these subtle messages that seem to emerge during social occasions can be very stressful. When combined with having no clear plan of how to navigate the situation food wise, this can lead to either overeating at the event or starving yourself at the event and then losing control of your eating as soon as you return home.

Why is this? Because in addition to the identity messages you are already navigating, when you starve yourself at a party you may also be adding messages of deprivation and injustice subconsciously to your inner dialogue, such as, *"It's not fair,"* and *"everyone can have some but me."*

Over and over I hear from members that after denying themselves completely at a party or restaurant, they found themselves self-sabotaging after they arrived home. So that begs the question— what stands out with the members who are successful in social situations?

Two things I have observed. They eat along with everyone else, and they have planned ahead. In other words, they have created enough margin in their lives to check ahead that the food has low-carb and sugar-free choices, or they have brought along some delicious food for themselves. This also means that there should be a larger layer of planning going on at home.

U = UNDERSTAND YOURSELF

Nothing is more defeating than opening the fridge during a time of hunger only to find nothing to eat. So I coach my members to shop every week around the time of our weekly class while their weight-loss focus is high. I encourage them to buy ingredients ahead of time for making low-carb treats and give themselves the gift of creating enough margin for a prep time once a week.

In addition to this, you will need to do some research on where to eat when you go out. With a little bit of research ahead of time, you can know before you even walk in which foods are low-sugar/low-carb friendly, even at fast food restaurants like McDonalds. (A Caesar salad, hold the croutons, and a grilled chicken breast).

I currently do this / I need to create margin for planning

4. Tackle the stressors head on

Don't remain a victim of circumstance. If finances are stressful, then take a course on financial management. If your kids are too hard to handle, take a parenting course or ask older successful parents whom you admire to coach you in your parenting. If your house is always a mess, read some books on decluttering and managing household tasks.

I read a book when I was a young mom that taught me how to break down all household tasks into small jobs that were written on 3x5 cards and divide them up among family members. That book, along with a good parenting course, took me from being a stressed out mom with a messy house (who felt like emotional eating, due to the stress of it all) to a calm mom, with kids doing their part of the chores, and a clean house that was easy to maintain by following the simple strategies in the book.

In other words, emotional eating is often triggered by ignoring these kind of issues that push on you every day. So a big part of resolving emotional eating is to identify the main stressors in your world and deal with them on purpose.

I currently do this / I need to tackle things head on

5. *Learn how to move out of reaction and into calm*

We cannot control the events around us, but we can control our responses to them. If we allow them to, stressful events can cause us to be pulled out of our place of peace and into a state of either fight or flight, which in turn can trigger emotional eating.

We need a skill set to help us navigate our reaction to negative events and people and to return to center where we are connected to God's peace and in a state of emotional rest.

Let's look at dealing with negative people. Their behaviors (whether it is a rebellious child or a rude shop clerk) can trigger the fight or flight response. We will need to have a skill set for dealing with them, and it may not come naturally to us. This is because in the same way that favorite family food recipes are passed down to us, so are family recipes for dealing with conflict.

It has been my observation that emotional eaters often tend to move into flight and avoidance of conflict, which in turn causes them to internalize the unresolved issue. They walk away from relational conflict with adrenalin and anxiety coursing through their body and, with nowhere to release it, they then turn to food.

The other way this plays out is with the emotional eater who responds to conflict by blowing up and losing their cool. This often pushes away the person who they have the conflict with, and the issue remains unresolved. The rift in the relationship becomes an elephant in the room, and so they too internalize the issue and turn to food.

I created the acronym CALM to help my members navigate people problems without aggression or fear. CALM uses biblical principles for communication that help us physically, emotionally, spiritually and relationally during an encounter with others. Let's look at it together and see how practicing this relational strategy can help you navigate confrontation and return to a place of peace and calm, which in turn will help you stay free from emotional eating.

U = UNDERSTAND YOURSELF

C = Calm down
A = Ask questions
L = Love/keep your love on
M = Make it right/mask off

C = Calm down

When someone upsets us, it causes a physical reaction. Adrenalin begins coursing through our bodies, triggering the fight or flight response, and we are probably not thinking at our best. In fact, many people describe their mind as freezing up and they are only able to think of how they would have wanted to respond later, after the incident is over and they have calmed down.

So this tells us something important. **Allowing your body to calm down before responding to the situation will always result in better communication and usually a better outcome.**

Take a deep breath, and let your body return to a peaceful state. Take time before responding, or ask for a few minutes if needed, and leave the room. Sometimes though, confrontations are in public, and you cannot leave. You can, however, learn to be your own internal coach, using some positive self talk to remind you of this acronym.

Coach yourself to calm down and take a deep breath and you will see the difference that this makes immediately.

Proverbs 15:1 A soft answer turns away wrath, but a harsh word stirs up anger.

A = Ask questions

We are used to shutting down and running away in stressful interactions, or becoming angry and attacking. Asking questions is neither running or fighting; it is clarifying. A lot of times, negative interactions with others are simply miscommunication and misunderstanding. Perhaps they are having a bad day, and it is not all about us. This is often the case. Perhaps someone has made a wrong assumption that needs clarifying. Examples of good, open ended questions that invite clarification are:

Are you aware that _____?

Sorry, but I may have misunderstood, can you clarify _____?

Can we talk about what happened _____?

What do you think about _____?

James 1:19-20 So then, my beloved brethren, let every man be swift to hear, slow to speak, slow to anger; For the anger of man does not produce the righteousness of God.

Proverbs 18:17 The first one to plead his cause seems right, until his neighbor comes and examines him.

L = Love/keep your love on

Danny Silk, the author, speaker and relationship guru, says that the goal of healthy communication is to create and protect connection. He teaches us to *"keep our love on"* by not assigning a negative motive to the person's actions. This goes hand in hand with asking questions. I often frame my questions with an opening that declares that I believe that the person did not act intentionally to cause harm. For example I might say: *"I'm sure it was not your intention, but are you aware that _____?*

I find that even if the person I am dealing with is in a terrible mood, giving them grace will almost always open up their heart towards me, and allow me to communicate about what is happening, rather than sending a negative judgment that will escalate into a confrontation, causing both of us to react with fight or flight. Jesus told us that if we approach in a judgmental attitude, it will come right back at us. But love will disarm even our enemies.

U = UNDERSTAND YOURSELF

Matthew 7:1-2 "Do not judge others, and you will not be judged.

1 Corinthians 13:7 Love bears up under anything and everything that comes and is ever ready to believe the best of every person.

M = Make it right/mask off

So often we do not ask what it will take to make something right, or do not communicate to others what they can do to make things right. We walk away with an unresolved issue because we were unprepared to request action or offer to take it.

Obviously our interaction with a grocery cashier will not go deeply into our emotions in ways where we need to be too vulnerable. In this case saying, *"I am sure it was not your intention, but you have placed my bread under all my canned goods in the bag. Could you please re-bag my order with a fresh loaf on top?"* is enough. You are calm, assertive, communicating respect and love, but asking for what you need. This type of interaction will rarely trigger emotional eating, because it ended in a place of healthy communication.

However, when we are in a deeper conflict, M still needs to stand for Make it right, but should also stand for mask off. Be real! Emotional eating is triggered by feelings and thoughts that have been stuffed down deep. If you have a friend who repeatedly arrives 20-30 minutes late when you have made a coffee date and leaves you standing outside the shop waiting, you will need to become courageous and take your mask off.

In order to make it right in this case, you will need to share the impact that their behavior is having on your relationship. You will need to communicate to them about how you are experiencing them. It takes courage to take off your mask and speak from the heart, but the results are worth it.

So using the steps I have already outlined, an example of how to take off our mask while still keeping our love on would be, *"You may not intend to be late for our coffee dates, but you have been repeatedly and when you do that I feel _____ (hurt, let down, rejected etc). Can we talk about why this is happening?"*

This is an example of using all of the steps above and opening up the communication even on a potentially difficult issue. Generally, when confronted, people will make excuses. But once again, you will now have an opportunity to be assertive and ask for action.

"In the future, this is what you can do to make this right." (Text me if running late, leave earlier etc) You may even need to let the person know what you plan to do if the behavior continues. *"I am just letting you know that in the future, I will leave if I don't hear from you."*

Doing this will complete your part of the communication equation and allow you to walk away, knowing that you did your best, whether things are successfully resolved or not. You will be able to return to your center more easily when you have been honest about what's going on inside of you.

One more thing. What about when you are the one who is in the wrong? Let's go back through the **C.A.L.M.** acronym and look at the steps you can take when you have been accused of wrongdoing. I will reiterate here that the requirement for a small misunderstanding in public is much less than the requirement of making right a major offence you have committed towards someone close to you.

Always keep the depth of vulnerability appropriate to the depth of the relationship and you will navigate this successfully. Saying simply, *"I'm sorry"* is usually enough in small situations. Polite apologies and a smile are appropriate in public. Tears, careful listening and repentance belong to those we walk closely with.

HOW TO DEAL WITH THINGS COURAGEOUSLY WHEN YOU ARE IN THE WRONG

C = *Calm down*

This still applies. You need to navigate the issue in a calm state, free of anger and defensiveness. If you immediately feel angry and defensive, take a deep breath, and center yourself. If you're really angry, ask for a moment and step out and then come back to talk.

A = Ask questions

This still applies. Ask several questions to determine why the person thinks you have behaved wrongly. Ask them how they experienced it. Even if you have done nothing that you can see as wrong, if the person felt wronged by you this is your opportunity to help them find freedom from being upset and offended. Ask them clearly, *"How did it make you feel when I did that?"* When I follow these steps, This information moves me away from defensiveness and anger and helps me understand what I have done to offend.

L = Love/keep your love on

When I have been the one to cause offence, my job is to communicate to the person I am speaking to that I value them, and that I value our connection. I want to let them know that I want to keep our relationship because of the value that I place on it. Communicating a loving commitment to ongoing connection turns a confrontation into a deeper conversation about your relationship. It is amazing how quickly anger and fear leaves the room when a commitment to see things through has been released. So by simply stating at the beginning of the conversation that you value the relationship, and that you are there to make things right, you will lower the anxiety in the room immediately.

M = Make it right/mask off

When you have wronged someone, it's fairly simple. After hearing how the person experienced the situation, simply saying, *"I am so sorry that you felt that way,"* or *"I'm so sorry that I did that,"* are appropriate responses. However, in a deeper relationship we may need to add, *"What can I do to make this right?"* It takes courage, but it's simple. You own your mistakes. You will almost always walk away after asking what you can do to make something right with a good inner feeling, low stress and low desire to emotionally eat. This is because your question invites the other person to engage in a dialogue about how you can build and restore the relationship.

That's the C.A.L.M. acronym. A healthy relationship recipe that helps you navigate conflict, rather than over-reacting or stuffing your emotions. It's easy to remember, because the word itself is the first step.

Having a good recipe for conflict is a big part of having a skill set for immediate issues that lead to emotional eating, but sometimes the stress we are experiencing is not people, it's events. Let's face it, tyrants and toddlers are not always willing to listen to reason, so we need to have other stress reduction skills in place. The following list of solutions and skills help to reduce the fight or flight response when you find yourself in situations that are stressful and that you have little or no control over.

Exercise

Your body experiences exercise as fighting back. It drains off adrenalin and other stress hormones, and boosts your feel-good hormones. Fifteen minutes of exercise will do this for you. A brisk walk, a bike ride, whatever gets you moving. Your body will interpret the exercise as having dealt with the threat to your wellbeing, and your desire to stress eat will be lower.

A hot bath, a warm heavy blanket or other change in environment and temperature

Occupational therapists know that wearing a weighted vest helps to settle a hyperactive child by calming the central nervous system. We can do the same thing with a hot bath or heavy blanket. It seems a bit silly to picture it, but the principle works. Calm the central nervous system and you lower the fight or flight response.

U = UNDERSTAND YOURSELF

Prayer

Turning the problem over to God will help you to enter into emotional rest by releasing the emotional issue before it becomes buried in your soul. Practicing forgiveness while issues are small is a healthy spiritual practice. I would like to suggest that you combine prayer with either a walk or a hot bath, because that will give you the advantage of treating both the physical stress and the emotional stress that you may be experiencing.

Connection with others

When you cannot resolve an issue, for whatever reason, whether it is an event beyond your immediate control, or a relational situation that defies your attempts to navigate it, talking over the issue with a friend can bring you into a greater place of emotional rest. Sometimes wise counsel is given, and sometimes it's just the sharing of the burden that lessons it. Either way, stress will be lowered and isolation will be broken, both of which are triggers for emotional eating.

Avoiding trigger locations and situations

A trigger is an association that causes a fight or flight response and can include places, time frames, people and things. This stress management technique helps you to head off food temptation before it even happens by recognizing the places, times, people and things that trigger you.

Stress eating often occurs in the same place, with the same foods, and at the same time of day. This causes powerful associations towards overeating to develop. To use this tool, make note of the places and times that usually trigger overeating. Plan your time differently so that you are not re-creating that set of triggers every day.

For example if you usually sit in a certain chair every night and overeat while watching TV, make a decision to read in your bedroom with a cup of tea during the evening. Or if you always give in and order junk food in a certain restaurant, then you need to make a firm decision to stay away from that restaurant as it is a place that triggers you to overeat.

Avoidance in all of these cases is both wise and strategic. This is especially important when we are feeling more vulnerable for whatever reason. We need to learn to understand ourselves and observe the negative patterns in our lives that cause repeated emotional eating. Once you recognize the pattern, you can make different choices in order to diffuse it.

This also applies to people. There are people who have either hurt us in the past, are hurtful now, or people we have a hard time saying no to. (Grandma and her special dessert that she makes just for you.) Being passive when around these people allows them to guilt us into eating or trigger old wounds from the past. There are some relationships that we may need to avoid for a season, limit time spent, or set firm boundaries for the times we need to interact with them. Heading into a situation with one of these difficult people is very different when you have prepared yourself. You can keep it short, bring a dish of food, and not allow their words or pressures to stick to you.

Finally, there are the things that trigger us. These are often foods that we have an old pattern of overeating or even dishes that we have used to overeat with (enormous bowls or plates). They can hold powerful associations with a loss of self control, because that's what happened so many times in the past.

We need to deal with stress the right way by keeping these foods out of the house and beyond arm's reach. We would not expect a recovering alcoholic to keep an open bottle of whiskey on his counter, and yet we can become caught in the trap of telling ourselves that we are keeping these foods in the house for our family or company, and then these foods are right there calling to us when we are feeling vulnerable. I like to challenge all of my EWL members to clean out the places and spaces in their lives by removing unhealthy foods, patterns, people and things. The Bible sums this up very simply in *2 Timothy 2:22,* "*Flee temptation.*"

U = UNDERSTAND YOURSELF

All of these techniques and tools above will help you to deal with the stressors and triggers in the surface layer of your life. That's right, we have only scratched the surface, and there are deeper places to look.

As I said in the first chapter of this book, the weight-loss industry does not even begin to address these many dynamics and the ways they impact us. So the good news is that if you have been stuck in your efforts at weight loss for years, taking the deeper journey through this book can release a whole new set of tools into your life. These tools can in turn offer you hope and a way to resolve emotional eating, just as they have for many others who have taken the Encounter Weight Loss course.

Now let's look a bit deeper to the other emotional layers that we discussed at the beginning of the chapter.

EMOTIONAL EATING
Part #2 Inner Attitudes

In the next layer, just below the surface of what is at the forefront of our minds, we find inner attitudes. This layer reveals what is really going on in our lives. It includes how things really are in our beliefs, in our spirituality and in our relationships with others.

It also includes our identity (not simply the things we have been told to believe about confidence and self esteem, but what we really believe about ourselves when no one is looking).

This layer may or may not be easily recognizable to us, but if we sit and think deeply, we can usually identify these beliefs. This is an important skill in dealing with this layer, because we need to connect honestly with our real feelings if we are going to understand ourselves in ways that will keep us free from over eating. I like to take time regularly to think deeply and ask questions like, *"What do I really want? What are my goals? How are my relationships doing? How is my connection to God?"*

The positive beliefs in this layer will not usually trigger emotional eating, but the negative and unresolved issues can. These are usually areas, where what we are feeling below the surface does not necessarily match the cheerful front we show on the surface of our lives. We could say that this layer represents us without our mask on. In this unmasked layer, there may be a lack of truly knowing our worth and identity, or a lack of satisfaction with an area of our life where we feel powerless to change things.

If we do not have a set of tools to deal with these strong emotions when they erupt, we may find ourselves emotionally eating. So the best tool for dealing with this under-the-surface layer is to take regular time to dig it up *before* it erupts!

At least once a week during my devotional/prayer time I ask myself some deep questions that help to keep this layer opened up. Here are a some questions that can help you navigate and identify your inner attitudes. Be willing to work though these questions in such a way that it moves you into a place of resolve about what you really want from life. You can develop action plans for your life and goals that flow out of answering these questions. Too often we just float along passively throughout life without ever addressing what is really going on under the surface, and the unconscious anxiety of these unanswered questions will fuel a desire to emotionally eat.

I encourage you to get a journal and work though the activation questions below, one at a time, day by day. That's right, answer one question per day. Don't rush through. Take the deeper journey and begin to uncover what's under the surface without rushing through. These questions will put you in touch with your own heart and help you to go deeper with God. God always invites us into an honest dialogue with him. Our foundation scripture for this chapter is: *Psalm 51:6 Behold, you desire truth in the inward parts. You teach me wisdom in the inmost place.*

So this tells us that He wants us to come to Him with all of our deepest questions and longings.

U = UNDERSTAND YOURSELF

ACTIVATION

I have grouped these questions under different headings that reflect the areas of our attitude and beliefs that can trigger emotional eating. Try taking one section or a few questions each day to think deeply about and journal.

How things really are

- How do I really feel about life right now?
- What parts of life am I content with, and which parts frustrate me?
- What gives me joy?
- What drains me?
- Do I have too much on my plate right now?
- Is there anything I need to do to reduce the pressure and expectations? (Delegate, say no, ask for help)
- Am I bored because I have nothing on my plate? No vision, dreams or plans?

Spirituality

- How is my connection to God?
- What would make it deeper at this time?
- Is there anything I am holding onto that I cannot simply release?
- Is there an area of my life where I am struggling to trust God?
- What events from my past are hindering my ability to live in the present? Do I need healing from them?
- In what ways is longing for an arrival at a certain goal preventing me from enjoying the journey?

Identity

- How do I really feel about myself, my identity, and self esteem? Is it positive? Or is it negative?

- If negative, where are the negative messages coming from?
- Who are they coming from? Who specifically have I given the power to determine my worth?
- In what ways am I hiding who I really am?
- What vulnerabilities am I afraid to share with others who love me?
- Is there any way in which I feel that I am not deserving or worthy?
- In what ways am I holding back love for myself?
- Do I need to gain some healing in the area of my identity?
- Where and how am I going to do that?

Status of relationships

- Is there anyone I need to forgive?
- Am I getting too caught up in other people's problems? Whose?
- How can I gain some distance?
- How do I allow other people to cross my boundaries?
- Where do I need stronger boundaries?
- What relationships require more of my time and nurturing?
- Am I prioritizing money, work or material things over relationships and my values?

Personal growth

- What do I feel passionate about, and how can I spend more time on my passion?
- How could I be more engaged in life?
- Where do I need more learning or skills?
- What would my friends and family say are my strengths?
- What would my friends and family say are my weaknesses?
- How does my work reflect my passions, skills, and interests?
- What would a beautiful life look like to me?
- What is stopping me from getting it?
- What would need to change to align me with what I desire?

U = UNDERSTAND YOURSELF

- What am I leaving unfinished that needs my attention?
- What is my vision for the next five years?

Self-defeating patterns

- Are all of my habits and actions positive and life giving? Which ones are not?
- If they are not positive and life giving, do I understand why am I doing that habit or action?
- What need do I think it is meeting? What would be the healthier way to meet that need?
- What (or who) am I tolerating that I really shouldn't have in my life?
- What negative thought patterns do I have consistently?
- How am I mistreating my body or compromising my health?
- What do I allow to distract me from really living?
- Are there any ways that I am being irresponsible or unwise financially?
- What foods does my body not react well to? Are there any that I need to cut out completely?
- Which places, spaces, people and things trigger me to overeat?
- What would be my best strategy to avoid or navigate these triggers?

Generational patterns and beliefs

- Am I living a life someone else has defined for me? In what ways?
- What are some patterns/sins that I see coming down the generations in my family? Are they affecting me? My children?
- Am I actively seeking help to break these patterns? If not, then why not?
- What expectations do I have for my kids that are more for me than them?

- In what ways do I want to be different than my parents?
- Do I need to let go of any belief systems to get there?

Deeper questions about life
- If I died tomorrow, what would I regret not doing?
- What legacy am I leaving the world after I'm gone?
- What legacy would I like to leave?
- What do I believe about eternity? How do I feel about this?

Once you have taken time to journal through these questions (this can take some time), I highly recommend reading the book called *Necessary Endings,* by Dr. Henry Cloud. In it, he provides a framework for bringing non-satisfying roles and relationships to an end. This can be a big help in deciding how to respond to some of the things you discovered just below the surface. There may be some roles and relationships that need to end in order to bring about a greater joy and satisfaction in your life.

EMOTIONAL EATING
Part #3 The Deepest Layer: Wounds And Trauma

In the deepest level of our soul are beliefs and thoughts that I call the beasts in the basement. These include deep emotional hurts, betrayals, losses, trauma, deep disappointments, and damaging identity messages that we have carried with us for a long time.

These issues are locked down in our soul, either because we won't forgive them, or we have tried to forgive them but the pain re-emerges unexpectedly. Like a sleeping dragon, these issues can come roaring to life and definitely cause not only emotional eating, but can also derail our long-term freedom in our weight-loss journey if we do not do what it takes to resolve them.

So let's look at some longer term, preventative strategies for our emotional health that will address the unconscious issues below the surface in our lives that keep triggering us again and again.

U = UNDERSTAND YOURSELF

Developing an skill set for dealing with deeper issues

This is the stop on the weight-loss journey where many people get off. Just as the deeper issues within us are often hidden and unconscious, our reaction to dealing with these issues can often be a subtle form of avoidance.

It breaks my heart when I see members of my weight-loss class avoid this stop in their journey, because I know that in order to truly resolve the roots of overeating, they will need to deal with some of these issues. When they are avoiding this step, they will suddenly become too busy to attend classes, and will often double their efforts at a quick-fix solution, which will eventually lead to a crash and derail their attempt to lose weight.

It takes courage to connect with others; it takes courage to open up, and it takes courage to deal with the past. It may seem easier in the short term to avoid the issues, but in the long term the reward of working through our issues is a life free from emotional eating, and a life full of new-found confidence. Resolving deeper issues involves both forgiveness and unhooking from negative identity messages.

We will discuss identity messages in our next chapter, but first let's conclude this chapter with a look at what it means to forgive.

Forgiving from the heart

Deeper issues are almost always rooted in an inability to forgive from the heart. We all want to be able to forgive. We have all likely heard the quote, *"Unforgiveness is like drinking poison in the hopes that the other person will die"* and various other statements made to motivate us to forgive, but I have personally observed that our willingness to forgive is usually not the problem.

Rather it is a lack of finding a forgiveness that goes beyond our head and all the way into our heart. We may have attempted to forgive in the past by doing what I call *throwing a blanket of forgiveness over the issue*. We make a surface attempt at forgiveness that does not connect with the deep pain in our hearts, the power of the trauma we experienced, or the vows and judgments we have made about ourselves, our life and others.

I have spent most of my career as a leader and pastor in the church, running emotional healing classes and doing one-on-one counseling, where I have the privilege of walking through people's traumatic and painful past issues with them. Through these many experiences, I have come to believe that revisiting the place of wounding and powerlessness from your past by telling your story, and giving an account of the deep pain you experienced, is often the key to unlocking forgiveness from the heart.

In the Bible there is a story that Jesus told about forgiveness in Matthew chapter 18:21-35. I have included it here for you.

21 Then Peter came to Him and said, "Lord, how often shall my brother sin against me, and I forgive him? Up to seven times?"22 Jesus said to him, "I do not say to you, up to seven times, but up to seventy times seven. 23 Therefore the Kingdom of heaven is like a certain king who wanted to settle accounts with his servants. 24 And when he had begun to settle accounts, one was brought to him who owed him ten thousand talents. 25 But as he was not able to pay, his master commanded that he be sold, with his wife and children and all that he had, and that payment be made. 26 The servant therefore fell down before him, saying, 'Master, have patience with me, and I will pay you all.' 27 Then the master of that servant was moved with compassion, released him, and forgave him the debt.

28 "But that servant went out and found one of his fellow servants who owed him a hundred denarii; and he laid hands on him and took him by the throat, saying, 'Pay me what you owe!' 29 So his fellow servant fell down at his feet and begged him, saying, 'Have patience with me, and I will pay you all.'30 And he would not, but went and threw him into prison till he should pay the debt.

31 So when his fellow servants saw what had been done, they were very grieved, and came and told their master all that had been done. 32 Then his master, after he had called him, said to him, 'You wicked servant! I forgave you all that debt because you begged me. 33 Should you not also have had compassion on your fellow servant, just as I had pity on you?' 34 And his master was angry, and delivered him to the torturers until he should pay all that was due to him.

35 "So My heavenly Father also will do to you if each of you, from his heart, does not forgive his brother his trespasses."

In the story, Peter asks him how many times we need to forgive. He was thinking that seven times seemed like a good number. Jesus responded *"No, not seven times, but seventy times seven times."* He then went on to compare forgiveness of sin, to the forgiveness of a debt, and said that we need to forgive from the heart.

We tend to skip over the details of the story and pressure ourselves to *"forgive or God won't forgive us."* Yet by looking a little deeper into this story, we can see a key to unlocking forgiveness within our own lives. That key is that our heart is like the man who had money owing to him. He took an account of all that was owed. Our heart is like an internal accountant. It gathers evidence against others for the wrongs we have suffered, and stores that evidence in the form of pain within us. This suppressed pain pushes up from our heart whenever we are triggered, such as when something happens that causes an association or memory of the pain. It's like our heart cries out, *"Wait, he still owes you for that!"*

In the story, the man who was wronged gave an account of what was owed to him, and this is the key. Again and again I have seen that as I sit down with someone and go through an account of what has happened, letting them tell their story and give the pain over to Jesus, something unlocks for them. God's Spirit ministers to them in ways that no amount of logic or positive self talk can achieve.

As time is taken to give an account, inner vows and judgments are often recognized and broken and the fuel driving the inability to forgive dries up. It is always humbling and an honor to walk through this with people, and it is truly a key to resolving emotional eating once and for all.

Below I have outlined some steps to help you take the deeper journey into forgiving from the heart. If you feel that you need help and resources beyond the range of the steps outlined below, I would recommend the ministry called Restoring The Foundations: www.restoringthefoundations.org

They have an amazing ministry that uses biblical tools to heal the pain of the past. However, I have outlined below some simple steps to emotional healing that you can work through with a friend. To do this successfully, review the steps below and plan a day where you can meet. My recommendation is that you only work on one person's issues for that day, and plan a second full day for the other person. This leaves lots of time for support during the healing session and processing time afterward.

Steps to emotional healing and forgiving from the heart

#1 Find a trustworthy person to walk with you through these steps. Choose someone who is in a journey towards wholeness themselves and who is comfortable walking through these steps with you without judgment or advice giving. A person who understands and practices confidentiality. Ask yourself if you are comfortable revisiting every scene from your past with this person.

#2 Set aside enough time for ministry. Plan an afternoon or evening to dedicate to this time of ministry so that you are not rushed.

#3 Pray together with your friend, inviting the Holy Spirit to reveal the hidden pain in your heart. Ask Him to bring to mind the names of people who He wants you to deal with and make a list of those names. Make sure your parents are on that list even if it does not seem necessary. Even the best parents can wound their child, so that relationship should be examined. Once you have received the names, then start at the top of the list with the first name. Ask the Holy Spirit to bring back to your mind the painful memories that need healing.

#4 When a memory scene comes to mind, give an account of the memory to your friend and to God. Tell the story, describe the scene, and identify the pain it caused. Give an account of your feelings of betrayal and sadness, rejection, abandonment, or other ways that you felt violated.

Use *"I felt _____ when you did _____* statements to take ownership of your emotions and feelings. You can do this by expressing the things you were unable to say and confront at the time of the offence.

Picture a chair across from you with the offender sitting in it and speak to the person as if they were there. After you have identified your feelings, end by reclaiming your voice with a statement like, *"I wish you would have _____"* Allow God to connect you with the inner pain until it is released. Have your friend or counsellor take notes about what you are sharing.

#5 Ask God to bring to your mind any vows or judgments you may have made during the event that happened. These will often be revealed during the time of giving an account described above. They are usually *"I will never"* or *"I will always"* statements about yourself, and *"You will always, and you will never"* statements about others. For example: An inner vow could be, *"I will never trust anyone again."* A judgment could be, *"Men will always leave me."* Once you have identified these vows, have your counsellor or friend write them down.

#6 Ask God if you believe any lies about yourself or life in general because of the event. Pray, *"God please show me any messages that this event sent to me about myself and life."* Some negative identity beliefs and messages may come to mind. Also ask God if you have believed any lies about Him? Tell your friend or counsellor about the lies that come to mind and have them record these.

#7 You have now taken an account of all of the fallout from this incident. Just like the man in the parable, you have listed all of the results of the offence against you, and in a sense what your heart felt you were owed for justice. Picture a bill with an accounting list of offenses on it. What are you going to do with the bill? Instead of trying to extract payment from the person who owes you, you are going to present the bill to Jesus.

Now forgive from the heart, presenting the list to Jesus and turning the burden and pain over to him. Ask Him to remove the trauma from your body and soul.

Next take the list your counsellor or friend has been recording and break agreement with all of the vows and lies that were revealed during the account you gave. Ask Jesus to redeem what has happened and to speak to your heart about how He feels about you. Wait before God together as you ask Jesus to speak to your heart.

This whole process allows God to replace the lies, vows, and wounding with His peace. Only God can be God and do this. Forgiveness from the heart occurs when we exchange our bitterness for God's peace and acceptance. It does not let the offender off the hook with God; it simply unhooks us from the pain of the event and opens us up to finding new hope and redemption from what has happened.

So you can see from exploring this chapter how important it is to your success to understand yourself. To understand the places, people and things that trigger you. To examine your heart and discover whether you are truly happy with life. To learn to build more margin into your life and to understand exactly what you need in order to be successful. Whether that is learning to understand what you need in a social occasion successfully, or who you need to forgive in order to heal the wounds in your soul.

Making the commitment to understand yourself, and take the steps through the activations in this chapter, is the biggest gift you can give yourself in resolving emotional eating and finding permanent lifestyle change. It is truly worth the journey.

UNDERSTAND YOURSELF — MY STORY

In 1996 I found myself sitting around a table in a small back room in my church with a group of twelve women. Everyone was nervous, especially me, and you could feel the tension and anxiety in the atmosphere. I had volunteered to lead an emotional healing group for women in order to help them deal with their emotional baggage from their past.

The irony of this situation was that I was likely the most emotionally broken person in the room. Talk about the blind leading the blind! I still smile when I think back to that day. Yet God had seemingly chosen me for this task to help other women find emotional freedom.

In looking back, I can see that as I cut a swath towards freedom for myself, many were indeed following me. I started that class by using another author's book as a guideline to help, but soon moved past it and began to write and teach my own material within a couple of years.

Along the way I took every inner-healing, emotional-healing and self-help course for confidence that I could find, eventually coming to the understand that there is not one perfect course or perfect answer to heal people's emotions and identity. Rather I was in the process of filling up a spiritual toolbox with many different tools that could be pulled out to help others as needed.

I found in time, that as long as the format or tool being used connected the person to Jesus, then healing would come. My own journey towards emotional healing from my wounded past contained the same steps I have outlined in this chapter for you.

I remember clearly the first time I created a list of names of the people who God was asking me to forgive. The list was very long and contained so many different people who I had encountered in my lifetime. From my grade school teachers, to my parents, it even included people whom I'd had short but devastating encounters with that had scarred my identity along the way.

Like the comedian who performed during the intermission of my cousin's dance recital, and decided to point me out in the audience and make me the butt of all of his jokes. It was only a short encounter, but the messages sent to my fragile ten-year-old self resulted in enormous emotional pain and some inner vows such as, *"I will never call attention to myself in public."* This eventually became a big hindrance to my destiny as a public speaker. But God was truly faithful to me, and over the years I continued to allow Him to clean out the pain, emotional freedom truly came to me. I went from being an out-of-control emotional eater who thought about food as soon as I woke up, to being able to keep food in the place it belongs in my life.

Along with the emotional healing work that I did in my own life, one of the tools that I shared in this chapter that was a real breakthrough key for me in my journey was the understanding of being triggered by places, people and things. I began to realize that I had eating rituals that occurred in the same way and in the same place and time every day. I had to learn to stop sitting in the same chair, and watching the same TV shows at night, because I had an eating ritual attached to that.

I had to let go of watching TV and move into my bedroom with a book and a cup of tea in the evenings in order to break the hold of that ritual. I also learned the hard way not to go past or into certain restaurants, and not to bring ice cream into the house. Ever!

To this day, although I have been free from emotional eating for a long time, if I bring ice cream into my house, I will have a very hard

U = UNDERSTAND YOURSELF

time not overeating it. There is just too strong of an association with self comfort and binge eating from my past. I have given myself the gift of only eating ice cream rarely and always outside of my home.

Another key that really helped me to break the cycle of trigger associations was to create new rituals each day that became strong positive associations with healthy living. I learned that the first one or two choices that I made in the morning could have a big impact on my day. What do I first put into my mouth, and what do I do first in the morning? My first choices would send a message of whether or not this was going to be a day of healthy choices.

By creating a ritual of eating the same healthy thing every morning, I began to send my mind the message, *"You are in control of your eating today; you are going to make awesome choices today."*

I learned to lay out my breakfast the night before, so that what I would eat was already decided when I got up. I began placing my Bible under my favorite coffee cup next to my coffee maker, which helped to remind to make take time for me and God along with my coffee every day. I was already trained to drink coffee every morning without fail, so by simply attaching a new habit to the established one, I was able to add in a positive new ritual.

The other key breakthrough for me in the area of understanding myself was when I came to understand that stress and anxiety are very physical and not just intellectual. I learned that I could lower my stress and anxiety with physical exercise. In fact, I learned that my body would interpret my exercise as me having successfully fought off or run from the threat. So I was now harnessing the idea of fight or flight in my favor. The physical part of the anxiety would be drained off, so the desire to numb the pain would dissipate.

The final key that slipped into place in my life in terms of understanding myself was when I finally began to get a handle on what I needed for social occasions and eating out.

I realized somewhere along the way in my journey that I had a subtle idea of being on or off my program. The picture I would use to best describe the way I viewed this is that I was like my dog, patiently walking along on a leash until we would get to the dog park, at which point I let him off the leash. This triggers him to be wild and crazy and disobedient, because he doesn't have a lot of skills to control himself, and so he only behaves well on the leash.

Well, I realized for myself that eating at home was like being on the leash, because I had everything very controlled there, and so there were not a lot of unhealthy foods to choose from or temptation or unexpected stressors, so I did fairly well. But once I hit a party or a restaurant, just like my dog without the leash, I would lose control. I would tell myself before I left the house that I would make a good choice, but it would seem that all good sense would go out the window once I hit the restaurant or party.

So I needed to conquer this one, and personally the way I did that (and this may not work for everyone) is that I learned to settle the matter before I left the house. I now decide exactly what I am going to eat before I leave, and I make sure that it is something that I will really enjoy, even if this means spending a little more on a dinner out or spending more to bring a delicious low-carb item to a party. Then I mentally rehearse seeing myself ordering and eating exactly what I have planned and I do that several times, leading up to the event. Once I get to the event or restaurant, my choices feel more like a well-rehearsed script than a moment of temptation. It took a while, but I did come to understand myself and you can find your understanding too!

I started this book with the question, *"If you currently use sweets and junk food to deal with your emotions, then how are you going to deal with your emotions when you give up the food?"*

It is my hope that this chapter has given you some tools that will help you answer that question.

References:

Dr. Richard Swenson, *"Margin: Restoring Emotional, Physical, Financial, and Time Reserves to Overloaded Lives"* (Oct. 11, 2004)

Chapter Eight

N = NO GUILT, NO SHAME, NO PERFECTIONISM

Isaiah 43:19 Behold, I will do a new thing; now it shall spring forth; shall ye not know it? I will even make a way in the wilderness, and rivers in the desert.

If we are going to see ourselves as people who are capable of being successful in losing weight and keeping it off, then the inner dialogue that we have with ourselves will need to be examined and, if necessary, the script rewritten. This is because we will never rise above the inner image that we have of ourselves. This inner image can color our self view so strongly that when we look into the mirror we will be affected by this inner view more than the actual image that we see.

This can result in a situation where we may have lost weight on the outside, but we still feel unattractive or worthless on the inside. This negative self view can sabotage our weight-loss efforts by acting like a default setting that causes us to return the exterior of our lives to match the negative inner view that we have brought with us from the past.

ENCOUNTER WEIGHT LOSS

ACTUAL EXPERIENCES
- At goal weight
- Weight varies within a five pound range
- Body is thinner
- Others say you look attractive
- Following program 90% of the time
- Has many friends at EWL

NEGATIVE SELF IMAGE

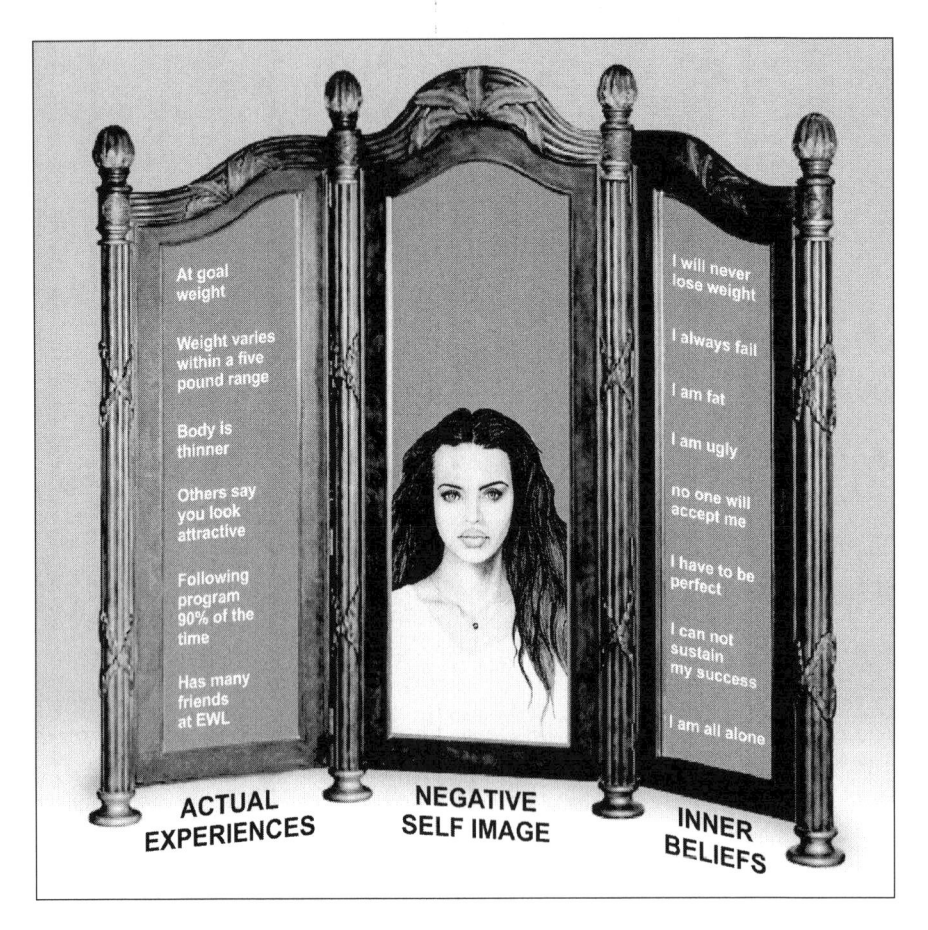

INNER BELIEFS
- I will never lose weight
- I always fail
- I am fat
- I am ugly
- no one will accept me
- I have to be perfect
- I can not sustain my success
- I am all alone

This inner image that we carry can be likened to an old suitcase full of *limitations* and *labels* that we have carried with us through life. When we come to look in the mirror, it's like we bring this baggage with us and paste these limitations and labels from our past onto the mirror. Then no matter what we have accomplished in our current life, these limits and labels are still with us and are still speaking to us every time we look in the mirror. They can act like a magnet pulling our attention into the past and denying us the right to enjoy our success or to be a different person than those labels and limitations dictate.

The key to removing them is to do two things. The first is to work through the forgiveness activation that I shared with you in the last

N = NO GUILT, NO SHAME, NO PERFECTIONISM

chapter. That is a powerful first step to becoming truly free. By forgiving from the heart, we remove the sting and fuel from the words and experiences of our past, but unfortunately that's where most people stop.

They do not understand that letting go of the pain is not enough. We must also take some powerful steps to re-frame our future by limiting the power that we give to people and experiences to attach negative identity messages onto us. That's right. We need to learn something very simple but very powerful. *"I do not allow what happens to me, to be me. I do not build my identity on my past, my performance, people's opinions, my possessions, or my position."*

All of these P's are subject to change and are an unreliable way to build your self esteem. They trap us into a cycle of guilt, shame and perfectionism as we try to use them to gain approval, acceptance and self esteem.

Let's break this down a little more:

When I build my self esteem on my performance, I only feel good when I am doing things perfectly. I can become trapped in a cycle of trying hard to be perfect, followed by crashing and giving up because I cannot sustain perfection all the time.

This can be especially true when it comes to weight loss. We can try to build an exercise routine that is based on never missing a day at the gym, or try to have such rigid control in our eating that it's all or nothing all of the time. When we live this way, a bad day or week where we make some wrong choices can totally derail us. We can feel unable to get back up and reconnect with healthy choices, because we are gripped by guilt and shame. This is all a result of building our identity on performance and perfectionism.

The same kind of cycle can happen when we try to gain self esteem through possessions or a position we hold. The perfect clothes, the perfect house, the perfect party, the perfect children, or whatever other perfect image that we try to achieve. Our sense of self esteem only lasts as long as everything is perfect. Of course since life is not perfect, when we build our self esteem this way, it comes crashing down whenever we cannot keep a perfect image in place.

What about people's opinions? Who have you allowed to tell you your own worth? Have you ever thought about the fact that a baby is born as a blank slate in terms of self esteem? A baby has no knowledge of her value or worth. These things are spoken into her along the way. Sadly, when we allow people's opinions to be the source of our self esteem, we are at the mercy of how people treat us, the things our parents spoke to us, and the negative dialogue that we carry with us.

When we build our self esteem this way, we can be feeling great about ourselves, and then something as simple as an encounter with a grumpy grocery clerk who treats us badly can allow a negative self esteem message to stick to us, one which we cannot seem to shake off.

So none of these ways is a reliable way to build your self esteem as they are all subject to change and lead to a cycle of guilt, shame and perfectionism that keeps us from real freedom. If we are going to move away from this, we will need to understand how to unhook from these negative cycles and messages that have held us back in the past.

We will do this in three steps:
- Exchange perfectionism for a lifestyle of grace
- Create a hierarchy of authority for validation
- Practice positive self-talk

#1 Replace perfectionism with grace

The first step is to break free from perfectionism as a source of self esteem. The reality of the cross should be at the heart of all we do. It should be at the center, and somehow we seem to walk by grace in all other areas, but when it comes to weight loss people try to accomplish it by rule keeping and law. By trying hard, then giving up, then trying harder again. By shame and guilt and trying to be perfect.

I like to use a unique example to demonstrate what it means to lose weight by grace, rather than law.

N = NO GUILT, NO SHAME, NO PERFECTIONISM

I have an elliptical trainer that measures my pace when I run on it. It has a message that comes up whenever I am running within ten paces on either side of the optimal pace for my height and weight. A light comes on and a message begins to flash that says, "pedaling in range.... pedaling in range... pedaling in range." It's like the machine knows that it's impossible for me to stay at the perfect setting for an extended period of time and so it sets a range for me to aim at, and as long as I stay in the range I am getting most of the benefits.

That's what the grace of God is like. You get the benefits that Jesus bought for you with His death and resurrection, even though you can only walk in the "range of holiness" without being perfect all the time. There is something about grace, about not having to be perfect, that takes the pressure off and allows us to make fewer mistakes than when we have the pressure of trying to be 100% perfect.

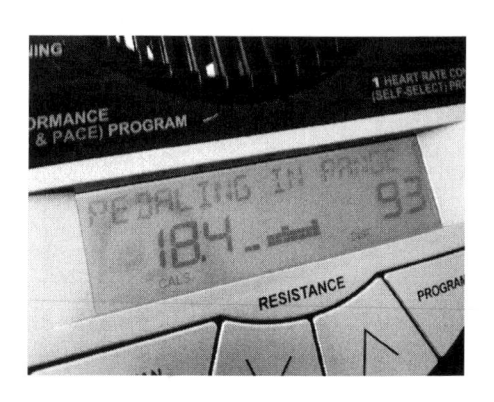

Walking by grace unhooks us from the identity message that we are a failure when we make mistakes. In fact, we have a saying in our Encounter Weight Loss groups called "feedback, not failure." This means that when we make some poor choices, we do not engage in messages of guilt and shame. We forgive ourselves, and receive God's forgiveness, and then begin to ask God and ourselves questions about what was going on that led to our poor choices. We look for feedback, life lessons, and information about our patterns and choices that help us understand ourselves.

Walking in grace when it comes to losing weight does not mean that we cast off restraint and don't care about the consequences. We still do our best to make good, healthy choices at every meal. Walking in grace speaks to how we respond when we fall down. Do we grovel in the dirt, or become full of shame, guilt and anger? Or do we apply the grace of God and quickly move into forgiveness and then observation and feedback about what happened? This second process begins to build confidence within us as we discover that we can come back to a pursuit of a healthy lifestyle.

I teach my members that guilt, shame and perfectionism are the enemies of weight-loss success. When I say guilt, I do not mean conviction by the Holy Spirit that leads us to repent. I mean the kind of guilt that remains even after repentance. A shaming guilt that sends an identity message that you are a bad person. Whenever we see guilt, shame and perfectionism in our life they are like a red-light warning system that tells us we are disconnected from the love of God. That we are gaining our identity from performing and trying to control the number on the scale though our own performance.

I teach my members to reject this kind of lifestyle, and to not meditate on or tolerate messages of guilt, shame or perfectionism that come at their minds. Rather, I teach them to step intentionally into grace, be gentle with themselves, forgive themselves, and embrace the imperfection in life by reminding themselves that they do not need to have it all together in order to feel good about themselves. This new way of thinking is enhanced by practicing our next step, creating a hierarchy of inner validation in our lives.

#2 Create a hierarchy of authority for validation

As I said at the beginning of this chapter, a baby is born as a blank slate. She has no opinion of her identity or self-worth, which is largely spoken into her by a variety of other sources. These sources include her life experiences and the messages she receives from her family, significant people in her life, her culture and the media.

It is easy to see that you could take the same baby girl and place her in two different homes, one which was loving and positive and one which was negative and abusive, and she would come out with a very different identity and level of self esteem. That is where the problem lies. When we build our identity and self esteem from these sources, we are at their mercy. If people tell us we are worth something then we

N = NO GUILT, NO SHAME, NO PERFECTIONISM

are; if they don't tell us we are not. Or if the media says that a size ten body makes you beautiful and you are a size twelve, then you do not meet the definition of beauty.

In order to break free from this, we need to ask the question, *"Who has the right to tell me what I am worth? Who decides what my value is? Who has that authority?"*

We need to learn not only to question this, but also to make a choice to create a hierarchy of validation in our life where we choose which people we give the right and authority to speak to our worth.

I want you to picture a pyramid. That's what a hierarchy is: it's a pyramid with the people who you allow to influence you at the top, and the people who should have no influence and authority to speak into your life at the bottom. So the answer to, "Who has the right to tell me what I am worth?" is actually determined by you! You give people the right by what you allow to influence and stick to you. Once you understand this concept, you can become very slippery and the labels and limitations that used to cling to you will have no ability to stick any longer. So let's look at how to create a hierarchy of authority for inner validation.

Who should be at the top? Very simply God should be at the top.

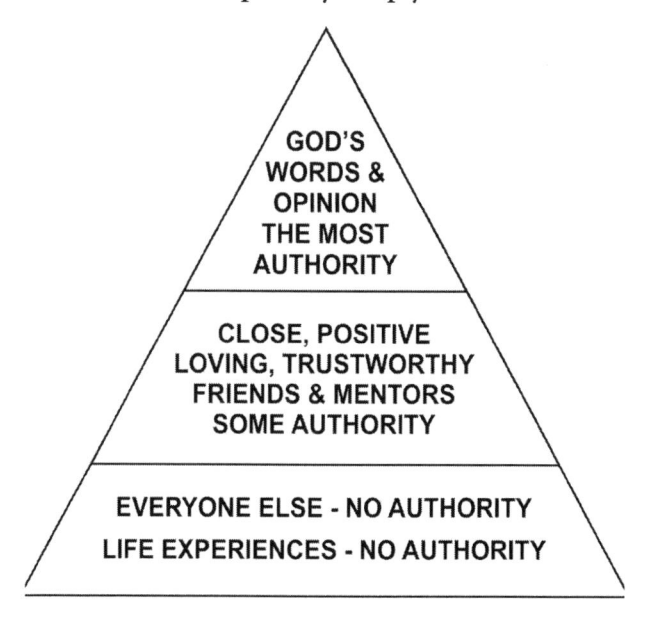

```
            /\
           /  \
          / GOD'S \
         / WORDS & \
        /  OPINION  \
       /  THE MOST   \
      /   AUTHORITY   \
     /─────────────────\
    /   CLOSE, POSITIVE  \
   /  LOVING, TRUSTWORTHY \
  /    FRIENDS & MENTORS   \
 /       SOME AUTHORITY     \
/───────────────────────────\
/   EVERYONE ELSE - NO AUTHORITY  \
/  LIFE EXPERIENCES - NO AUTHORITY  \
─────────────────────────────────────
```

God: the most authority to speak to my identity/top of the pyramid

His word is true. He cannot lie. He never changes. He says many powerful and wonderful things about us in the Bible, and His words should be the foundation for our self esteem and displace the negative messages we have allowed in. We can learn to do this on purpose by creating an internal hierarchy where we pull down negative messages and establish God's positive ones within us.

Close, positive, loving and trustworthy friends/mentors: some authority/middle of the pyramid

We need to surround ourselves with positive and uplifting people. People who believe in us, and who cheer us on in our journey. These are the people whose words should have value and authority in our life. A simple test is this. Do I feel good about myself and feel built up in my faith and vision for the future when I walk away from this person? Do they speak the truth to me in a way that is loving even when it is something difficult to hear? If a person meets this criteria then you choose to let them take that position and speak into your life.

Everyone else: no authority speak to my identity/bottom of the pyramid

Our journey towards wholeness requires some change in our relationships. When people have been negative, abusive or broken our trust, we do need to forgive them, but we also need to set healthy boundaries in place. If someone does not build me up or speak positively into my life, I intentionally limit their influence over me. Picture moving them to the bottom of the pyramid of influence. That is where they belong. This is also where the grumpy grocery clerk and the angry driver who just cut you off belong. When you understand this concept, you become slippery, because you have intentionally limited the authority of the words or actions of these people, so they have little ability to attach identity messages to you.

N = NO GUILT, NO SHAME, NO PERFECTIONISM

Life experiences: no authority to speak to my identity / bottom of the pyramid

The other thing that belongs at the bottom of the pyramid is life experiences. I like to say: *"I do not allow what happens to me to be me."* God's promises and his words over us are not based on our performance or circumstance and they never change. Therefore when I build my identity on His words and promises, I build it outside of my performance, my successes, my failures or any tragedy that comes to my life.

When I fail that failure does not become my identity, because God says that I am not a failure. When I succeed, I know it is not by my own strength, but by the grace of God and so that does not add anything to my identity which is already positive in Him. When unexpected circumstances or tragedy visit my life, I can hold onto the truth that God is always good, always loves me, that every good and perfect gift is from Him, and that tragedy and evil do not come as a message from Him.

That's right, tragedy is never a secret message from God to hurt me, punish me or make me feel worthless. The scriptures are clear that God is love and a redeemer of this fallen world. So I limit the right of my circumstances to send any identity message to me, so that I can boldly say, *"I do not allow what happens to me to be me. I am who God says I am, and I am worth what He says I am worth, and that is totally outside of my circumstances."*

#3 Use positive self-talk

Our final step in this core value is to learn how to implement positive self-talk into our lives. God has given us the ability to frame up our future with our words in the same way that a builder would frame up a house in the shape he wanted it to take on. The scripture shows us that God framed the world with His words:

> *Hebrews 11:3 By faith we understand that the universe was framed by the word of God, so that what is seen was not made out of things that are visible.*

ENCOUNTER WEIGHT LOSS

Genesis 1:3 And God said, "Let there be light," and there was light.

This is a word planet. It was created by words spoken out of God's mouth, and when we speak words that are in alignment with God's word and opinion about us, we enter into that creative process as well.

My observation is that there is an overcoming power available to us, through the words we speak, and that in the same way our negative speaking in the past has kept us bound, positive speaking can set us free. It can release creative power to cause our thinking and health to come into alignment with our words. I personally believe (and science is showing) that our cells hear the frequency of our words, either positive or negative, and vibrate with the frequency they hear, either producing sickness or health, powerlessness or confidence. So our words are an important part of our path to wholeness, and when we speak out decrees in alignment with God's words, this brings His empowerment into play.

The Bible says in : *Job 22:28 "You shall also decree a thing, and it shall be established for you: and the light shall sign on your ways."*

This is a great scripture that describes what happens when we begin to speak positive words over ourselves. The thing we are speaking becomes established in us, and the path to walk it out opens up in front of us. Think of it as an exchange. Purposely cast down and limit the negative voices, opinions and thoughts have been a part of your past, and exchange them for new positive statements that frame up your future in the same way that God framed the world with His words.

I encourage you to tackle positive self-talk on several fronts. First begin to speak more positively all the time. Begin to talk success, freedom, healing, and overcoming. Say things like, *"This time I am staying with my weight-loss journey until I get to my goal weight,"* and *"I am changing all the time, this is working for me,"* or whatever other positive words come to mind.

N = NO GUILT, NO SHAME, NO PERFECTIONISM

Catch and correct yourself whenever you find yourself speaking negatively or from performance with words like should and have to. Guilt, shame and perfectionism are not only the enemies of weight-loss success, they are also toxic to us in many areas of our lives. Walking free from these ways of thinking and behaving is an essential part of our weight-loss journey. In addition I want to encourage you to learn to intentionally speak out decrees over your life during your prayer time. We will do this as our activation/encounter for this lesson.

NO GUILT, NO SHAME AND NO PERFECTIONISM — MY STORY

I grew up with very low self esteem. My family was not demonstrative with affection or words of praise. So in the absence of any positive information about myself, I believed the worst and allowed guilt and shame to speak louder to me than any other voice in my world.

I was born in the 1960s and came of age in the early 1980s during the birth of the internet, with its sudden parade of unrealistic body sizes and "perfect" models being held out as the standard that we should all long to achieve. I could not deal with the expectations or meet that standard, so I developed an eating disorder (bulimia) by the time I finished high school. This became compounded by perfectionism and striving to keep everyone happy, which in turn led to stuffing my feelings of self-rejection and wearing a mask all of the time.

It was a long road for me to learn how to limit the power that I gave to others to define me, and yet here I am in my 50s, so much more confident and free than I was in my 20s. And why? Simply because of God extending His grace to me, in giving me His identity and worth as conveyed through the scriptures.

And God didn't just give me a new identity, He taught me to break free from the power of guilt, shame and perfectionism by intentionally creating a hierarchy of authority and removing the old limitations and labels I had allowed to be placed on me along the way.

I can't express how important this is, because at the core of the journey we are studying here is our Encounter with God who wants to love us as a person in process. Not a person performing, not a perfect person, but a person in process. For me this meant that I could let go of my ideal weight and the number on the scale as my goal, and enjoy the journey and process towards greater health overall. I now think of a goal range rather than a goal weight, and health and longevity are my main focus.

I have learned over the years that shame and a fear of being vulnerable are the two greatest barriers to freedom that we carry as humans. So as we shed these barriers, we begin to soar in ways that we were limited in up to this point. We open up, we begin to take risks and we move from a constant stream of negative and self-accusatory dialogue in our heads and into a place of feeling cherished and at peace.

This has been the journey for me and it has changed the core of my weight loss journey from "I have to do this because I hate myself" to "I want to do this because I love myself." And in this, I have experienced true transformation from the inside out.

ACTIVATION

I have included some positive decrees for you to declare over your life. I encourage you to practice being slippery by creating a hierarchy of authority with people's words and actions, while at the same time decreeing these new statements over yourself. Do this during your personal prayer time and whenever you have a negative encounter with a person where you feel like your self esteem has taken a hit. I have included space for you to write some of your own decrees that counter some of the specific negative messages you have carried with you in the past. Write a decree that declares the opposite of the negative message that has been with you. Now declare success and freedom.

If identity and self esteem have been ongoing struggles for you, then I would like to recommend my teaching course called *Looking*

N = NO GUILT, NO SHAME, NO PERFECTIONISM

Beyond the Mirror, which contains an in-depth study of identity and self esteem, and takes you on a foundational journey to rebuild your identity from the ground up using biblical truth. It is available at www.wendypeter.com

VICTORIOUS DECREES

Write these words on 3x5 cards or read them from this book and declare them over your life.

- I am made in the image of God, and in the name of Jesus I decree that my body is conformed to His likeness.
- I decree that my body is a temple of the Holy Spirit, and day by day it is becoming a fit habitation for the indwelling presence of God.
- Jesus has healed every area of lack, insufficiency and insecurity in my life; therefore, I decree there are no empty places within me that I need to fill by over eating.
- I do not worry about what I shall eat or drink. My heavenly Father will always provide everything I need.
- Jesus is the bread of life; therefore, I decree that He satisfies my every desire.
- I decree that my metabolism is supercharged with the power of Heaven and I have abundant energy and strength.
- I decree that my spirit, soul and body surrenders to the Holy Spirit and brings forth the fruit of patience and self control.
- I decree that I am no longer a slave to fear; I am not bound by the enemy and I am bold as a lion. I am a child of the King, and I stand as a powerful child of Heaven taking dominion in my body and in my life.
- I decree that I will successfully lose all excess weight, regain my health and be a testimony of the saving power of God to all I see.

ENCOUNTER WEIGHT LOSS

Now add a couple of your own specific decrees.

Chapter Nine

T = TAKE BACK YOUR DREAMS

Proverbs 29:18 Where there is no vision, the people cast off restraint.

I believe that food addiction and obesity steal our dreams and our destiny in God. I have seen again and again that those who struggle with obesity slowly move from being a participant in the center of life, to being a spectator along the side lines. Or as one woman put it, *"The bigger I got, the smaller my world became."*

God never designed you to be a spectator, to be shut down, uncomfortable in your own skin, afraid or embarrassed to participate in life. He designed you to be fully engaged, to be a dreamer and an influencer with a voice. Think back to when you were a child. The freedom you had as you participated with life and the dreams that you carried. God wants to restore those dreams to you, and connect you to your greater purpose so that you can live your best life.

In order to do this, we need to re-connect with our hidden dreams and receive fresh vision from God. Because without a greater sense of purpose, our weight-loss issues can keep us as a spectator and also cause us to give up through weariness or apathy, because we lack a compelling enough reason to get to our goal.

The Bible says in Proverbs 29:18 *"Where there is no vision, the people cast off restraint."* I like to say it this way: *"There has to be a more meaningful reason for you to lose weight than a number on the scale or a dress size."*

You see, without a connection to a larger purpose, losing weight becomes an endless pursuit of the world's values and validation that is tied to a number on the scale and that's simply not enough. Deep down we know we are meant for more than that, and I want to take this chapter and help you learn to tap into your gifts and activate your dreams.

Have you ever thought about the fact that God needs a vessel to carry His dreams? He cannot do anything in this world without vessels to move in and through. Yet so often we are quick to disqualify ourselves from God using us. We think, "what can I do?" We imagine that we will require an extraordinary level of talent and unique ability, when in reality God only needs a willing vessel. He only needs our *"yes"* and He will provide the assignment, the alignment and the resources to carry out His dream through us.

I love the story of Mary when she had her encounter with the angel of the Lord before conceiving Jesus. In the first chapter of Luke, the angel appears to Mary and tells her that she has found favor with God, and will conceive a son. When Mary asks, *"How can this be, since I am a virgin?"* The angel replies, *"The Holy Spirit will come upon you, and the power of the Most High will overshadow you;"* (Luke 1:35)

In the same way, the Holy Spirit comes upon us and the power of God overshadows our weaknesses when we give our simple yes to God. This is because we are called to live supernatural lives, to be carriers of God's glory. People are unhappy and unfulfilled because they are full of everything but the dream of God, everything but His purposes. They fill up on food and worldly pursuits as a substitute for living out of the dreams and purposes that God has designed us for. In other words as the Bible says, *"Without a vision, we cast off restraint."* *(Prov. 29:18)*

T = TAKE BACK YOUR DREAMS

Jesus observed that the unbelievers were obsessed with the issues of food and clothes and then challenged His disciples to *"seek first the Kingdom of God and His righteousness, and all these 'things' will be added unto you."*

Matthew 6:31-33 So don't worry about these things, saying, 'What will we eat? What will we drink? What will we wear?' 32 These things dominate the thoughts of unbelievers, but your heavenly Father already knows all your needs. 33 Seek the Kingdom of God above all else, and live righteously, and He will give you everything you need.

In other words, He challenged them to get into an alignment where they were pursuing their God dreams first, and then all of the other things would come into the right place and alignment in their lives.

So how do we come into this alignment with God's dreams for us? How do we rediscover that part of ourselves that has been shut down? How do we become a spectator instead of a participant?

My experience in working as a pastor in a church has taught me that as humans, we often complicate things that God meant to be very simple.

We imagine that a dream from God would need to be extreme, outlandish and involve great amounts of money and travel. While that may occasionally be the case, I believe that overall God wants to use us just as we are, in our current life circumstance, right now, today. In the same way that He came to Mary and asked her to yield herself just as she was to the purposes of God, so our Heavenly Father looks for us to partner in His dreams just as we are. Yes, just as we are, with the same personality, place and position of influence that we have right now. This offering up of what we have, to His divine purposes, is what I call the seedbed (soil) that God will grow His dream out of. Because very simply: God's dream, placed in the garden of my life, if watered, will blossom into a fruitful destiny.

Let's take a look at the seedbed that we can offer up to God right now. Answering these simple questions is really the first step to taking back your dreams.

#1 What am I good at?

When I am activating people in their dreams I always say, *"I want everyone to think of one thing they are good at and it does not need to be spiritual."* When I do this people come up with everything from cooking, to writing, photography, carpentry, counseling, listening to others and a multitude of other things they are good at.

Everyone is good at something, even those who think they are not good at anything, and even those who society might think have little to offer.

In the Old Testament story of the Exodus from Egypt, when Moses told God that he didn't think he had what it took to save the Israelites, God responded by simply asking, *"What is in your hand?"* Moses replied, *"A staff."* It was a shepherd staff, the tool Moses was already used to working with. God began with what Moses had in his hand, that which was familiar to him, and he eventually became the greatest leader of the Old Testament.

#2 How can I offer this to God?

Once people identify what they are good at, I like to activate their inner dreamer (which has often been shut down) by asking two questions. The first is, "Are you using that thing that you are good at to help build God's Kingdom?" The second is, *"If not, then what activity can we think of that will allow you to use this gift to build the Kingdom?"*

I have had wonderful brainstorming sessions with many people as we take something simple like a talent with sewing or photography and talk about the many ways that that gift can be yielded to God as a seedbed for His dreams. One young man decided that he would have a social evening open to anyone who wanted to come, where he would serve coffee and show them some basic things about photography. In

T = TAKE BACK YOUR DREAMS

brainstorming this dream, we quickly realized this would be a great way to reach out to people who were not comfortable stepping into a church on a Sunday morning.

Another lady who is not very mobile is sewing covers for some prayer mats we use in a prayer center in our church.

#3 Where did I give up participation that I need to take it back?

Sometimes taking back your dreams is literally just that, reclaiming something that you gave up somewhere along the way because of your weight problem. Somewhere that you can see that you moved from being a participant into a spectator. This can be anything from riding a bike, to wearing shorts or a bathing suit, participating in a social function or taking a vacation.

There is an old Christian song that goes *"I went to the enemy's camp and I took back what he stole from me..."* and sometimes that is simply what we need to do. Think back to your childhood and younger years. What were some of the activities that gave you joy? Where did you give them up along the way? It's time to take them back.

Every step we take like this exercises our inner dreamer and is an important part of our encounter with real change. A couple of years ago, I took back the simple joy of bike riding, by purchasing a vintage-style bicycle and beginning to take short rides with my husband on Sunday afternoons. It may look like a small victory on the surface, but it was a piece of the larger picture of my healing and taking back what I had lost to being overweight and injuries along the way in my life journey.

What do you need to take back from the enemy's camp? You will get a chance to answer that question in the encounter activation at the end of the chapter.

#4 Can I gain a higher sense of purpose by planting a stop sign somewhere for God?

Once we learn to offer ourselves up to God as a willing vessel for Him to plant His dreams in, we will find ourselves stirred to a higher sense of purpose in His Kingdom. When our heart is open to the dream giver, He will often give us an increasing sense of justice and show us how we can make a difference in the world by standing up for specific issues that move His heart.

As we practice using our gifts in ways that serve God's Kingdom, our boldness will increase and we will be able to move with God against the injustices in our realm of influence. Whether that means feeding the poor, visiting the sick, helping a single mom, or working to free women and children who are being trafficked throughout the world. Every small thing we do for God allows Him to move through the world, with us becoming the literal hands and feet of Jesus.

This was brought home to me three years ago in a very real way when I found myself going up against city hall in my home town in a fight to have a four-way stop sign installed on a very busy, dangerous street next to a children's playground. I do not consider myself to be very politically minded, so it was very out of my comfort zone to hand out fliers, make a presentation at city hall, and speak to news reporters. Yet the compelling of God was there within my heart and I came to believe that God was using my actions to save some specific lives that would have been taken by the many accidents happening along that road.

Now whenever I drive along that road, I come to "my" stop sign and I am reminded that God has called each of us to plant a stop sign wherever He asks us to, whether that is on a physical road for safety or a moral road where we work to push back the darkness by displacing it with our light and love. When we become vessels to carry God's dreams, we often find ourselves deciding to stand up in our generation and say, *"not on my watch"*, while evil things happen. Where can you plant a stop sign that will make the world a better place? This kind of activity pulls us up into a higher connection with our purpose and engages us in God's Kingdom in very real ways.

T = TAKE BACK YOUR DREAMS

#5 How does this bring my weight-loss into context within my dreams?

I started this chapter by saying that food addiction steals our health and our destiny by keeping us trapped as a spectator in life rather than a full participant. I also said that there needs to be a greater reason than a number on the scale or a dress size to lose weight. As we learn to take back our dreams and become a vessel for God to work through, the motive for our weight loss will shift and come into alignment with God's plans for our life.

The new and better *reason* for me to lose weight is to be able to have the stamina and strength to accomplish the God dreams that I have been given. I can unhook from my identity being tied to a number on the scale and become lost in the joy of being a vessel that God is using in amazing ways both big and small.

If my dream is to go on a mission trip, then I will need to be able to fit in a plane seat, step into a boat, climb a hill and eat whatever is set before me. If my dream is to use my skills locally to help others, then I need to be able to do my task with confidence and stamina as I work with others. If my dream is to be there for my kids and grandkids, then I need my health to be strong and have the mobility to get down on the floor and play with them. If my dream is to travel, I need to be able to move through space confidently and sit in a variety of spaces for longer periods.

All of these dreams can and should feed your weight loss vision, so that your higher purpose becomes something that you begin to pursue in which weight loss is a necessary component rather than a vain goal unto itself.

#6 How do I feed my dreams and accomplish them?

Once you begin to dream even in small ways, it's like turning on an inner switch. You begin to dream everywhere. There is an empowerment in knowing that all God needs is your willing yes, and He promises that He will overshadow you with His power.

However, if we were to read in detail Mary's encounter with the angel, we would see that God *waited* for Mary's yes before He overshadowed her. He waited for her important words. *Luke 1:38 And Mary said, "Behold, I am the servant of the Lord; let it be to me according to Your word."* So God waits for our yes to His desire to dream through us, and that is the first step to feeding your dreams.

Simply give God your yes: your permission for Him to use your life as a vessel for His dream. In addition to this, I would encourage you to do any of the following steps from this lesson's activation encounter that will build and feed your dream.

TAKE BACK YOUR DREAMS — MY STORY

I have already shared several stories throughout this chapter about the ways that I took back my dreams through things like getting back on a bike and stepping out to fight injustice. However, at the core of the deepest dream that I wanted to take back was the desire to regain my health because God had a call on my life to travel the world and preach the gospel.

My health was in the way of that dream, because I was suffering from such serious chronic pain from my old injury on my left hip and leg that I could not sit comfortably for more than 20 minutes, and sleeping in a strange hotel bed was an exercise in sleeplessness.

When I first cut all sugar and refined carbohydrates out of my diet, I did not cheat at all for the first year, and the changes in my health were dramatic. The inflammation in my left side reduced by over 50% and I could comfortably sit during the day. I began to sleep better at night and the horrible bouts of all-over inflammation where every joint would flair up also disappeared. I took up exercise and began to stretch out my left side and strengthen those muscles that had been weak. I felt great and I was celebrating having taken back my health.

Then came the second year. It started slowly, a little cheat here and there and telling myself, "It's no big deal, I'm still thin." Unfortunately, that was not the case. I was becoming too inconsistent with insulin

T = TAKE BACK YOUR DREAMS

levels and the old symptoms came creeping back.

So I found myself facing a decision. "How badly do you want your dream, Wendy? If you really want to travel the world, and if you want to take Encounter Weight Loss to all the people who need it, you are going to need to live it out every day of the year. No cheating, because while that may be OK for some who do not have your health issues, it will not work for you!"

Decisions, decisions.... I was in the valley of decision and I had to fight for what I wanted.

Well, as I write these words, I am sitting on an airplane coming back from a three-day conference where I just spoke to a group of women and coached them into *their* dreams. So I am happy to say that I made the right choice. I take back my dreams and my health every day with the principles God showed me for the Encounter Weight Loss course, and I have never felt better in my life. Beyond that, I have the joy of knowing that I am being used as a vessel for God's Dream for you...to help you be set free into a place of health and fulfillment yourself!

ACTIVATION

- Write down one or more things that you are good at.
- Take time to talk with others and brainstorm ways your talent could build God's Kingdom. Do this on purpose.
- Write down any dreams and activities that you have lost along the way to being overweight or in ill health, and identify what you need to do to take them back.
- Add to this list a few other dreams that you may have. (A travel dream, a financial dream, a ministry dream, a relational dream, a business dream, a material dream.)
- Set goals to take small steps towards the activation of each of your dreams. Even one step is a step closer to a dream.
- Make a vision board or scrapbook page that points to the dream. Keep this vision where you can see it when you pray.

If your dream involves missions or travel, hang up a map of where you are going and keep it before you.
- Be open to new ideas and big ideas. Those crazy ideas that you get in the middle of the night or those which seem to come out of nowhere are often the seeds of ideas that God wants to give us. Let your heart be a fertile seedbed for those ideas to land in and dare to dream big.
- Once you have identified a dream that you want to pursue, begin to soak it in prayer and map it out step by step. As you learn to partner with God in His dreams, you will see His faithfulness and provision for your dreams and find yourself living a life with true Kingdom purpose. Finally, keep the dream in front of you.
- Let your God dreams become really big, so that on the challenging days of your weight-loss journey, you have something bigger than a number on the scale or a dress size to pull you back towards all of the other core values that you have been pursuing. You will have a powerful reason to lose your weight that ties into God's greater purpose for your life.

Chapter Ten

E = EXERCISE AS A LIFESTYLE

1 Timothy 4:8 Physical exercise has some value, but spiritual exercise is valuable in every way, because it promises life both for the present and for the future.

At the risk of offending some, I would like to make a statement. I believe that exercise is one of those things (much like the pursuit of thinness in our society) that can become a bit out of balance. With a multi-billion dollar industry of equipment, potions and powders all designed to turn back the clock and promise eternal youth, somehow having six-pack abs and buns of steel has turned into a measurement of our success and value as people.

Two or three hours spent each day at the gym is now considered both normal and necessary by many, and those who don't buy into pursuing this perfect image are rather disdained. This does not mean that I am criticizing everyone that does this. I have friends who love pursuing fitness as a hobby, and they are also strong Christians who use their love of fitness and bodybuilding as a way to shine the light of God's love on the people in that community.

However, that is not the case for many people who can be found spending hours at the gym. Somewhere along the way, a twisted identity message has crept in, and external appearance has trumped inner beauty and character as the goal to be attained.

Yet the scripture here is simple. *1 Timothy 4:8 "Physical exercise has some value, but spiritual exercise is valuable in every way, because it promises life both for the present and for the future."*

So I would like to take this chapter to focus on the value of exercise without idolizing it in the way that the fitness industry has done over the last few years. And just to clarify, in my journey towards health and freedom, I too have done it all: bought the equipment, spent hours at the gym, and pursued the six-pack abs. But in all honesty, my motive in that time was to pursue a body shape more than health, and exercise was not in the right context in my life. So as I share these thoughts with you, I am coming from a place of learning to find balance and pursue health first rather than exchange my time and energy for the world's version of success and beauty.

My relationship with exercise has always been pretty much the equivalent of trying to get into a cold pool. Once I am in, I get used to the water, and even enjoy it, but it's the getting in that's the real challenge. I often end up in a mental battle, standing at the edge of exercising, trying to decide if I really want to go into it. So I cannot actually say that I love to exercise, but I love to be able to say *I have exercised.* Emphasis on past achievement as in already having accomplished the deed!

I have given a lot of thought to this seeming contradiction in my life, and I have come to realize that for the most part, exercise has had a lot of negative connotations for me and perhaps for others as well. Thoughts like…

- I have to
- I should
- It will be uncomfortable
- It will be too hard
- I'm too tired

E = EXERCISE AS A LIFESTYLE

- I have no choice but to do this to lose weight
- No pain, no gain

Added to this list are the images posted all over the internet of muscular, fit, super-athletic women running marathons or excelling in spin classes with six-pack abs. Those images always felt like an unachievable state of fitness for me to attain and provoked an ongoing feeling that no matter how much I exercised, I should always being doing more, faster, and better. So for most of my adult life I have gone through fits and starts of exercise, all propelled by the negative thoughts above and the world's motivation of wanting to be thin more than healthy, and the belief that exercise was a necessary evil I must endure in order to achieve that goal.

Imagine my shock when I was reading Gary Taubes' book, *Why We Get Fat, and What to Do About it*, I came to his statement that the scientific evidence to show that "exercise will make you lose weight *is less than compelling.*"

I went on to read multiple studies that all pointed to the same idea. Thermodynamics, as in "you must burn off more calories than you consume" is no longer the accepted explanation for weight loss and weight gain. In fact Taubes goes on to say that there was a time when virtually no one believed exercise would help a person lose weight.

Until the 60s, clinicians who treated obese and overweight patients dismissed the notion as naive. When Russell Wilder, an obesity and diabetes specialist at the Mayo Clinic, lectured on obesity in 1932, he said his fat patients tended to lose more weight with bed rest, "while unusually strenuous physical exercise slows the rate of loss."

The problem, as he and his contemporaries saw it, is that light exercise burns an insignificant number of calories — amounts that are undone by comparatively effortless changes in diet. In 1942, Louis Newburgh of the University of Michigan calculated that a man expends only three calories climbing a flight of stairs — the equivalent of depriving himself of a quarter of a teaspoon of sugar or one hundredth of an ounce of butter.

"He will have to climb 20 flights of stairs to rid himself of the energy contained in one slice of bread," Newburgh observed. So why not skip the stairs, skip the bread, and call it a day? More strenuous exercise, these physicians argued, doesn't help matters, because it works up an appetite.

Gary went on to say that his favorite study of the effect of physical activity on weight loss was published in 1989 by a team of Danish researchers. Over the course of 18 months, the Danes trained non-athletes to run a marathon. At the end of this training period, the eighteen men in the study had lost an average of five pounds of body fat. As for the nine women subjects, the Danes reported, "no change in body composition was observed."

This shift in perspective was a real challenge to my viewpoint on exercise. Take away the *"I have to do this to lose weight"* belief, and I was no longer sure what my motivation was when it came to exercise. Did I even want to exercise? Was there any benefit at all, given the fact that I now have the ability to maintain a healthy bodyweight by keeping the amount of sugar I consume to a low level?

These are all important questions that I have looked at and the answer is *yes*. There are many compelling reasons that exercise should be a part of your lifestyle, but they are not about achieving a number on the scale, rather they are related to overall health and longevity. These reasons carry a more compelling motive than "skinny" for exercising. Just as I said on our last chapter T=Take Back Your Dreams, there must be a greater reason for the changes we make in our lives than a number on the scale.

So let's take a look at the benefits that pursuing exercise as a lifestyle can offer, while at the same time moving away from the negative mindset that has seen exercise as a punishment to be endured by so many of us. Is it possible that we can re-discover exercise as play, a social event, or peaceful self care? Once we let go of our negative

E = EXERCISE AS A LIFESTYLE

framework for exercise, all these are possibilities. I have kept my summary of these thoughts brief, as the purpose of this book is to help you with the inner journey and a shift in motivation. So I would encourage you to read in depth some of the science referred to in my brief summary.

First of all let's look at four benefits of exercise outside of the old belief system of burning off calories. What does exercise really do for our bodies and our health? Here are a few powerful ways that exercise impacts us.

Longevity

Overall, regular physical activity reduces the risk of death by 30% in men and 42-48% in women.** This means that outside of what you weigh, physical activity will help you to live a longer and more active life.

How does exercise do this? In her recent book *Younger****, author Sarah Gottfried says that exercise alters the expression of thousands of genes thought your body, turning off some of the harmful ones, and turning on some of the beneficial ones. She goes on to list everything from insulin sensitivity and a decreased risk of cancer, to improved digestion, better cognition and a lower resting heartbeat as being positively affected by our genes coming under the influence of exercise. Rather than painting a picture of hours and hours spent in the gym as necessary to spark these changes, Sarah points out that most of these gene switches can be triggered by exercising three to four times per week for 30-60 minutes, such as brisk walking.

Detoxification

According to research reported by the Centers for Disease Control and Prevention (CDC) in 2005,***** more than 2,000 people tested showed traces of about 60 different toxins, including uranium and dioxins, in their systems. A sedentary lifestyle of sitting all the time and living in air-conditioned spaces can work against our body's ability to detox. We can improve the ability of our body to detox naturally through exercise. Movement stimulates the body, which stimulates blood circulation, which in turn causes sweating, increased thirst and greater detoxification through the kidneys and liver. With all of the toxins and chemicals that are in our world and affecting our food stream, this is an important part of protecting our health.

Mood improvement and stress reduction

Study after study has shown that exercise not only elevates mood, but it can also be as effective as medication for treating depression. When we exercise at even a light level, cortisol levels go down and feel good hormones like serotonin are released into our blood stream.

The fight or flight response that we experience as human beings (which I discussed in our chapter on emotional eating) when threat or danger is at hand comes into play here. Simply living in our world with its constant stream of negative news about terrorism and tragedy causes us a vicarious amount of stress and trauma that can have a negative impact on our health. I believe our body interprets exercise as fighting back (as in the fight or flight response) and this sends our body the signal that all is well and we have escaped the stressor, which then results in an overall lessoning of stress hormones in our body.

Exercise as play and social interaction

Children do not enter a playground with the thought, *"I need to burn some calories."* They enter the playground to have fun and spend time with their friends. In the same way, we can re-frame our experience with exercise to be a time of social activity and fun with others. This can include anything from bike riding or walking with a friend, to playing tennis or team sports. The social connection that is made during these times has a direct bearing on our physical and mental health.

Making exercise a lifestyle

So in looking at these benefits of exercise, it is not hard to see that while there may not be compelling evidence that exercise will cause

E = EXERCISE AS A LIFESTYLE

weight loss, there is compelling evidence that we should be exercising regularly to improve our health. So how can we motivate ourselves to make this change and bring exercise into its place as a normal part of our lifestyle? I would like to offer three keys after my story as an activation that I believe can help.

EXERCISE AS A LIFESTYLE — MY STORY

As I write this, I'm thinking back to the time in my life when I was the heaviest. At that time I had lost a lot of my mobility and exercise seemed unattainable for me on so many levels. It wasn't just the physical battle; it was the mental battle. I just felt too tired to exercise, and yet as I began to lose weight, a desire to move more was emerging in me.

So I began with walks, and I used those walks to pray and engage with God while listening to calming music. In looking back, I realize that I was tapping into many of the right motives for exercise without actually realizing it. Eventually as I walked and prayed, I began to envision myself moving even more. I saw myself running, even though I was not currently able to do that. Yet the desire was there. That was a turning point for me, because I had a moment of inspiration and thought to myself, I may not be able to run completely, but I could run for 30 seconds.

And so I began. Walk 30 seconds and run 30 seconds and eventually I worked up to doing this for 30 minutes. I didn't know at the time that I was actually doing something called wind sprints, which is a training style for runners. I was simply doing what I felt I could do.

My fitness level began to improve in leaps and bounds with the pattern I was following and eventually I added in stair climbing, once again just doing what I could. It wasn't until I was on a trip later that year in the Ozark mountains when I went out for a jog with a friend that I realized what had happened. I was actually really fit! I was leaving her behind huffing and puffing as we jogged through the mountains. My fitness level had increased to a level I had never imagined I would attain.

So the moral of my exercise story is simply start where you are, increase gently as God leads, and you will be surprised at how your body and your health change over time as you simply make exercise a lifestyle.

ACTIVATION

#1 *Put the fun back in*

If exercise has been a negative experience for you in the past, I would encourage you to only pursue fun exercise, at least at first. Re-framing exercise as play rather than punishment can make it into a totally different experience for you. It can help you to break free from the avoidance mindset you have held in the past.

Approaching exercise as play can also bring benefits to your relationships. In our busy society, people are finding it harder and harder to prioritize time with their friends and family. Exercise as fun allows you to spend relationship time with others. It can be very social and satisfying to play together. Look at the names of these activities below. Do any of them sound fun to you?

Circle the ones that sound fun, and start including them in your life without worrying about the frequency or intensity.

Aerobics, Ballet, Badminton, Baseball, Basketball, Biking, Boating, Bowling, Boxing, Canoeing, Camping, Dancing, Field Hockey, Football, Frisbee, Golf, Gymnastics, Hiking, Hockey, Hopscotch, Horseback Riding, Hula Hooping, Ice Skating, Jogging, Juggling, Jump Rope, Laser Tag, Paintball, Pickleball, Ping-Pong, Playing Catch, Rock Climbing, Roller Blading, Roller Skating, Skateboarding, Skiing, Soccer, Swimming, Tae Kwon Do, Tennis, Trampoline, Volleyball, Walking, Wall Climbing, Weightlifting, Wii Sports Games, Zumba

E = EXERCISE AS A LIFESTYLE

#2 Don't overdo it

One of the most common reasons people quit exercise is they take on too much too soon and cannot sustain the change. At the beginning of this chapter I referred to myself always having a feeling that I should be doing more, going faster, increasing my weights etc. This was usually a recipe for guilt, shame and perfectionism that kept a negative mindset in place and might have led to injury and burnout.

Paradoxically, when I began to pursue exercise as play and relaxation and I stopped driving myself to always do more, I became much more likely to desire exercise. My injuries went down, and I was more consistent in the long run. So start with a reasonable goal of once or twice per week that you can sustain and build from there.

#3 Find your exercise hook

We all have different personality types and reasons for pursuing the activities we find satisfying in life. What motivates one person to go to do something may not appeal to another person at all. Saying *"just do it" (Nike)* may motivate a person who thrives on a challenge, but will only cause a feeling of pressure and resistance in another. Over the years I have observed a few different things that will pull us towards exercise that flows into alignment with our personality type. I call these exercise hooks. They give us the extra pull that we need towards exercise. If you are not currently exercising, could it be because you have not found the right fit for your personality? Let's take a look at these four exercise hooks and see if you can find yours.

• For the intense leadership personality

This person likes achieving a goal, going further, beating their own record, competitive sports, and getting alone in nature to reduce stress. This personality often prefers to work out alone, and doesn't need others to motivate them, unless they are competing against that person. This person's exercise hook is a *personal challenge*.

- **For the structured planner personality**

This person likes planning exercise into their schedule, following a circuit at the gym, being part of a class, instructing others, and team sports with clear structure and rules. This personality loves to research and can fuel their desire to exercise by educating themselves on the latest research on the health benefits of exercise. This person does well with or without others alongside their exercise time and prefers to schedule exercise into their plan. *This person's exercise hook is scheduling and planning.*

- **For the creative, social personality**

This person loves to have fun. They love sports and activities that allow them to socialize and laugh with others while exercising, (volleyball, baseball, bowling or exercise that involves music like dancing or Zumba.) This person does best with people to exercise alongside of. *This person's exercise hook is socialization and fun.*

- **For the peaceful, calm personality**

This person is motivated by keeping harmony within themselves and everyone around them. They are good listeners, good friends and they don't like to rock the boat. They are very relaxed and by nature don't like to be excessive or out of control. They are usually drawn to exercise that reflects this, such as walking in nature, stretching, biking, swimming etc. This personality is also a very loyal and faithful friend. While they may not keep an appointment with themselves for exercise, they will never let down a friend. Therefore this person can activate their exercise hook by finding an exercise buddy to meet up with regularly. *This person's exercise hook is harmony and loyalty.*

#4 Take on an exerciser identity

The way we see ourselves has a powerful influence on our actions. An active person sees themselves as an exerciser. It is a part of their inner

E = EXERCISE AS A LIFESTYLE

life and identity. The way they plan their time and picture themselves doing life will include activity and movement. The way they describe themselves will be as active. We can help ourselves along in this part of the journey by beginning to intentionally change the way we see ourselves.

I remember when I first began to exercise and go to the gym. I definitely did not feel like *"one of those exercise people"*, as I used to refer to them. So I went out and bought myself some running shoes, an exercise outfit, and a special bag to organize my toiletries at the gym. It was an important part of changing the way I saw myself. I was giving some fuel to my desire for change.

It's funny, in looking back, I can see that obsessing about and buying all of the equipment was actually a part of avoidance of actually starting to exercise (*"I will work on all aspects of this going to the gym thing without actually exercising,"* was probably my unconscious thought). However, the day finally came where I had run out of things to buy and was all dressed up as an exerciser waiting for somewhere to go. And so I did go to the gym, and once I got there in my exercise gear, I actually began to exercise. So ask yourself, *"Do I see myself as active or not?"* Then think about some ways that you can embrace being active and healthy as a part of your identity in your speech, your dreams, your gear, and your choices.

#5 Make movement a lifestyle

Our final thought in this chapter is that exercise should become a lifestyle. I challenge my members to simply move more than before whenever they can. Once we get rid of the *"I have to exercise to move the scale"* mentality, we can begin to realize that every bit of movement we make counts towards good health and wellbeing in far different ways than simply losing weight.

That's right, everything counts. In her book, *The First 20 Minutes: Surprising Science Reveals How We Can Exercise Better, Train Smarter, Live Longer,****** New York Times bestselling author Gretchen

Reynolds addresses the issue of exercise as a way to improve longevity and happiness as well.

> "The first 20 minutes of moving around, if someone has been really sedentary, provide most of the health benefits. You get prolonged life, reduced disease risk — all of those things come in the first 20 minutes of being active," she said in a 2012 interview.
>
> "Two-thirds of Americans get no exercise at all. If one of those people gets up and moves around for 20 minutes, they are going to get a huge number of health benefits, and everything beyond that 20 minutes is, to some degree, gravy. That doesn't mean I'm suggesting people should not exercise more if they want to. You can always do more. But the science shows that if you just do anything, even stand in place 20 minutes, you will be healthier."

In addition, one study published in 2008****** found that those who exercised on work days experienced significantly improved mood on the days they exercised. Interestingly, while their mood remained fairly constant even on non-exercise work days, their sense of inner calm deteriorated on those days. According to the authors, *"Critically, workers performed significantly better on exercise days across all three areas we measured, known as mental-interpersonal, output and time demands."*

Key findings included:

- 72% had improved time management on exercise days compared to non-exercise days
- 79% reported improved mental and interpersonal performance on exercise days
- 74% said they managed their workload better
- Those who exercised regularly also reported feeling more than 40% more "motivated to work" and scored more than 20% higher for concentration and finishing work on time.

E = EXERCISE AS A LIFESTYLE

So if you are sedentary, there is hope for you. You can come out from under the all or nothing pressure to exercise and needing a perfect body that the media so strongly promotes. You can take back the joy and fun of movement, making it play instead of work and use it to build and honor your primary and important relationships with friends and family. You can increase your emotional well-being and your response to stress and improve your cognitive abilities. And you can increase your longevity by activating the genes that control aging and disease.

All by simply putting exercise in its place and making it a normal part of your lifestyle!

References:

** Samitz, G, et al., *"Domains of physical activity and all cause mortality: systematic review and dose-response meta-analysis of cohort studies"* (International Journal of Epidiology 40, no.5 2011)

*** Sarah Gottfried Younger, (2017)

*****Second National Report on Human Exposure to Environmental Chemicals January 2003 Department of Health and Human Services Centers for Disease Control and Prevention*

*****Gretchen Reynolds , *The First 20 Minutes: Surprising Science Reveals How We Can Exercise Better, Train Smarter, Live Longer*

****** International Journal of Workplace Health Management *2008* (ISSN: 1753-8351)

Chapter Eleven

R = RUN TO GOD

Mark 4:8 And other seed fell into good soil, and as the plants grew and increased, they yielded a crop and produced thirty, sixty, and a hundred times [as much as had been sown]

Woven throughout this program has been the thought that you need to invite God into your weight-loss journey. In fact that is probably the reason that many of you have purchased this book. You knew intuitively that the world's approach to weight loss was too shallow and that you needed to take a deeper journey. So it is fitting that we conclude this journey with our last core value **R=Run to God**, because truly it is the ability to learn how to turn to Him during times of temptation that will set the stage for long-term freedom from food addiction.

The Bible has a parable that Jesus taught that uses the concept of Satan uprooting a crop that was planted to teach people about the ways that we get pulled out of our dreams and lose sight of the promises that God has spoken in the Bible.

We can find this story in the "parable of the sower" that Jesus taught in Mark, chapter four. Read through Mark chapter four on your own, and then let's take a look at portions of it together…

Mark 4:3 "Listen! A farmer went out to sow his seed. 4 As he was scattering the seed, some fell along the path, and the birds came and ate it up. 5 Some fell on rocky places, where it did not have much soil. It sprang up quickly, because the soil was shallow. 6 But when the sun came up, the plants were scorched, and they withered because they had no root. 7 Other seed fell among thorns, which grew up and choked the plants, so that they did not bear grain. 8 Still other seed fell on good soil. It came up, grew and produced a crop, some multiplying thirty, some sixty, some a hundred times."

Jesus went on to explain this parable to His disciples by saying, "The seed in the story is the word of God which is sown into our hearts." So in the case of our weight-loss journey, the seed is the word of victory that God has given us to deliver us from overeating. It is the word of His promise for our success and freedom.

So with this context, let's look at the ways that Jesus said that Satan tries to steal our dream of victory from us. (The words in parenthesis are mine), and I have summed up each section with a D-word to point out three basic strategies that he uses in the story to keep us from the successful completion of our weight-loss journey. If we can learn to recognize these strategies for what they are and run to God whenever they happen, we will gain a lot of momentum that will take us successfully into the place of health we are seeking.

The first strategy: Doubt

Mark 4:14 The farmer [God] sows the word [of promise for victory from overeating]. 15 Some people are like seed along the path, where the word is sown. As soon as they hear it, Satan comes and takes away the word that was sown in them.

Notice that in the parable this seed was sown on the path and as soon as the people heard it, Satan came to take it. The path in this parable is the pathway of your thinking. His strategy of doubt comes at your thoughts as soon as you hear the promise of God for you to be

R = RUN TO GOD

freed from overeating, and tries to take away your promise. Doubt will come immediately at your thoughts with statements like, *"You can't do this, you have no self control."* It whispers things like, *"This won't work for you, don't even try."*

It tries to swoop in along the old pathways of negative thinking in our minds by magnifying our past failures. Our enemy tries to cause us to believe that his power to defeat us is greater than God's power to help us! He knows that if he can get us to doubt, we will give up trying to change our life before we even get started. At the first sign of temptation, he will use doubt to magnify how hard it is to change, how much we are going to suffer, and he will use these thoughts to try to get us off of God's promise.

Of course he reminds us of all the quick-fix starvation diets we were on in the past. He does not want us to think about the fact that we can now eat whenever we are hungry by simply choosing low-sugar healthy foods. He wants to make us associate weight loss with deprivation and failure, so that we will give up as soon as we start. He doesn't even need to activate his other strategies to get us off course, because this one has worked for him every time.

So how can we respond to this? We can simply recognize doubt for what it is: one of the hurdles we need to overcome in our journey. The Bible says that, *"All things are possible to him who believes." (Mark 9:23)* We can cut off doubt at its knees and run to God by magnifying God's ability to help us over Satan's ability to defeat us.

I like to challenge my EWL members to do this with a combination of scripture and positive self-talk. Jesus rebuffed Satan's attempt to cause Him to doubt in the story of the mount of temptation by saying simply, *"it is written"* and then quoting scripture. Have you ever thought about that? Jesus was tempted by food, and had to put it in its place just like you do. In fact, the scripture he used is a great one to start with.

> *Matthew 4:4 Jesus answered, "It is written: 'Man shall not live on bread alone, but on every word that comes from the mouth of God.'"*

Here is another scripture for dealing with doubt.

1 Corinthians 10:13 No temptation has seized you except what is common to man. And God is faithful; He will not let you be tempted beyond what you can bear. But when you are tempted, He will also provide an escape, so that you can stand up under it.

Now let's combine this with a self-talk strategy that I give my EWL members. I ask them to meditate on this during the first weeks that they are making changes in their lives and decree it over themselves, because it helps them to disempower the negative mindset they have held in the past. I have them practice a meditation that allows them to "doubt the doubter" and question Satan's ability rather than allowing him to question theirs, and to decree these scriptures over their lives, reminding themselves that this program is not about deprivation but about healthy choices and self honor.

I encourage you to write this on a 3x5 card and carry it with you. I recently showed my class a card like this that I carried with me in my purse for months, pulling it out whenever I was tempted. Here it is, for whenever you are attacked with the idea that it is too hard to lose weight…

"What if the truth is that it's not hard at all? What if it's actually easy for me to lose weight and change my health? What if it's just a deception that I have believed that I can't do this? What if I have been buying into the lie that it's hard and that's why it has always seemed hard? That's right; I decree in Jesus's name that the truth is this is easy and it will continue to be easy. This is easy for me because the all-powerful One is in me and with me! He has got this. He has got me! I can do this and I can choose this! I can change my life and my future, and right now, today, I am stepping into it this truth! I will not live by bread alone but by every word that comes from the mouth of God. I will not yield to temptation, but right now God is making a way of escape and showing me what healthy foods I can choose right now. I will do it!"

So we can defeat this first strategy of doubt and temptation by activating our faith on purpose and believing that we actually can lose our weight. We can reinforce this with scripture and positive self-talk.

The second strategy: Disappointment

> Mark 4:16 Others, like seed sown on rocky places, hear the word (of promise for victory from overeating) and at once receive it with joy. 17 But since they have no root, they last only a short time. When trouble or persecution comes because of the word, they quickly fall away.

Those words, *they quickly fall away,* could simply be translated as "they become disappointed and give up." Disappointment is the strategy that Satan brings against those who get going on their weight-loss journey very positively. They do not have the issue of doubt like the people in the first group. Many of us can lose weight initially and start out with joy as the scripture above says, but we get knocked out with the reality of taking the deeper journey and making the long-term commitment to change.

We can intellectually agree with the idea that a quick-fix is not the answer. But in actuality, after an initial few pounds are lost, the moment we have a setback we give up and become disappointed, rather than going deeper. So we remain in the words of the above scripture, *not deeply rooted.* We may have a hard time admitting that we need to give our commitment to a support group weekly and possibly long term for the times where *"persecution comes because of the word."* The persecution that comes against our weight-loss journey often comes in the form of family members not supporting us or peer pressure at social gatherings that brings temptation.

It takes time and accountability to learn to navigate these challenges, and if we have not committed to a regular and long term connecting with others, we will succeed only for a short time before quitting through disappointment in our amount of weight loss. Or we may, in the words of the above scripture, have trouble (also translated as anguish and inner pressure) that we need to overcome to take hold of our victory. This trouble, anguish and inner pressure may be self esteem issues or bitterness from our past that always rears its head again and again to steal our dreams.

Notice in the scripture above that the seed was sown on "rocky places". This symbolizes the state of our heart being hard, and the journey we need to take to soften it and open it up towards God, becoming rooted in His love and confidence in every area that we need it. So how can we deal with this strategy of disappointment?

We need to make a full commitment to the deeper journey, which in reality is a commitment to let God fully be God in an area of our life where we have not allowed Him to have full reign. This is in itself the essence of our journey into encounter with God when it comes to weight loss. It is said that whatever you turn to in a time of stress or crisis is revealed as your source. It is not hard to see that when we turn to food for comfort, stress reduction, entertainment, and friendship that it has become an idol.

Of course none of us wants that, but if we step back and look at our lives objectively, we can see that we learned to turn to food because of wounding or a lack of skills in dealing with relationships and stress, or because we were lonely and bored (which may be rooted in isolation and rejection or perhaps a lack of vision for our future.) All of these underlying causes of overeating are fixable with God, but we need to stay in the room with Him long enough for the fix, and we may need the help of others as counselors, coaches, and encouragers along the way.

I like to challenge the members in my classes to take other emotional healing classes that are tied to self esteem and identity (like my course *Looking Beyond the Mirror*), in addition to taking part in the healing and forgiveness encounters outlined in this book. This positions us to defeat this strategy of disappointment by facing up to our setbacks rather than allowing disappointment to knock us out before we complete our journey.

The third strategy: Distraction

Mark 4:18 Still others, like seed sown among thorns, hear the word; 19 but the worries of this life, the deceitfulness of wealth and the desires for other things come in and choke the word, making it unfruitful.

This is the strategy that comes against the achievers, those who have done well and made significant changes in their lives and who are on their way to victory. Those who are losing weight. The enemy knows at this point that he can't stop you, so he tries to slow you down by dividing your focus.

Let's face it, as I have just outlined, it takes some time and effort to make a permanent change in our lifestyle. If you have a significant amount of weight to lose, it can take a long period of time to cross the finish line. Along the way we can find ourselves at times just going through the motions. We know what we should be doing, and yet sometimes we find ourselves only doing it some of the time, because we have been at this for a while and it can be hard to maintain focus.

In the words of this scripture we get distracted, *"The worries of this life, the deceitfulness of wealth, and the desires for other things come in and choke the word, making it unfruitful".* It is true. We do have a lot going on in our lives and it is easy to allow the "desire for other things and the worries of this life" to creep in and distract us from having a razor-sharp focus on our health. And while this may not be enough to steal our victory, it can really stall us out at times and delay our progress. So I would like to give you some strategies that you can use to defeat distraction and cross your finish line in a timely manner.

Feed your focus

The first strategy in defeating distraction is to continually feed your focus. You can do this by simply subscribing to weekly email newsletters by doctors and nutritionists who believe in natural medicine, or about eating real food and the science of nutrition. Ongoing education will help to fuel your drive for change. Several of the writers and doctors I have quoted in this book have weekly newsletters that you can subscribe to. You can find their names in the resource section of this book. I find that whenever I pursue ongoing education about nutrition, my motivation to be healthy is sustained.

Don't make room for excuses

Distraction can keep us from pursuing the things that matter most to us, and then it's tempting to make excuses or become defensive about how we are doing with our weight loss. We can become lax, skipping accountability meetings and remaining vague about what we are eating. We may lose focus with grocery shopping and begin to eat out. I have found that the best resolution for this distraction from healthy choices is to be totally transparent in sharing with others about what is happening. This allows those on the journey with you to encourage you and challenge you in the ways that you need it most. Allow them to ask you the hard questions and regain your focus by strategizing with them about what you need to do to reclaim it.

Get involved

Nothing will keep you focused more than giving truth away to others. At some point in your journey, especially if you have a lot of weight to lose, it will help your focus to begin to help others in their journey. Share during meetings if you have access to them; start a support group if you don't. Volunteer to help others lose weight or even meet others to exercise. All of these things can help you increase your focus and take a stand against the strategy of distraction.

Maintain your intimacy with the Lord

God should be replacing food as your source. If you find yourself emotionally eating, don't beat yourself up about the food; simply go deeper with God. Intimacy with Him not only fills us up with love, but it also fills us with truth, and truth will sharpen us, keeping us from

R = RUN TO GOD

self-deception. Our spirit is made to rule in the house of our body, and our body is meant to be a slave to our spirit.

> *Revelations 5:10 says: And (He) has made us unto our God kings and priests: and we shall reign on the earth.*

So this is the way that God has created us to function. Your spirit should be ruling over your body and your body is supposed to be a slave to your spirit, but when you surrender to food, your body rules and your spirit becomes a slave.

Proverbs 19:10 sums this up saying: It is not fitting for a fool to live in luxury, much less for a slave to rule over princes.

We know intuitively that the desires of our body should not be running our life, but many times we make the mistake of trying to fight the desires of the flesh rather than simply running to God and cultivating a lifestyle of worship with him. Intimacy and worshiping God flips that equation around and brings your body under the rule of your spirit. It brings you into divine alignment, and instead of "fighting the desires of your flesh," you are now coming from a place of reigning as the "king and priest" of God that He has created us to be.

There is a wonderful promise in the book of *2 Corinthians 3:18* that says simply: *And we all with an unveiled face, beholding as in a mirror the glory of the Lord, are being transformed into the same image, from glory to glory, even as from the Lord, the Spirit.*

This is a wonderful analogy of the shift that takes place as we allow God to reign in our lives, creating a picture of us gazing into God as in a mirror (in the same way we used to focus on our body and all of our flaws). So now our gaze has come onto Him, with the promise that as we do this we are being *"transformed into His image"*. Intimacy with God is of course a lifelong pursuit, but in particular it is important for the emotional eater who has a past habit of keeping God out of that part of their life. As soon as you see the symptoms of emotional eating in your life, it is a cue for you to move in closer to God and allow Him to meet your emotional needs instead of turning to food.

I would also like to make note of the fact that we will never arrive at a point in life where there is nothing in us that needs adjusting. So, emotional healing should be a lifetime journey as well, and it's important to remain open to what God is saying. I personally went through some deep adjustments by the Lord in terms of my self-view once I had been at my goal weight for a while. I had been eating healthy for a long time and God wanted to break me free from tying my value to the scale. I did not think I did this, but then I sensed an inner prompting from God to stop weighing myself for a time, so I stopped.

After a month or two of not weighing myself, I had a sense of the Lord speaking to my heart one day and asking me if I liked my body. I looked at myself in the mirror that day and came to the realization that I had always tied my like of my body to a number on the scale. Now I no longer knew the number, and I had to answer the question outside of the scale. I realized then how much I actually had tied my self-view to a number on the scale, rather than a record of how healthy I had been eating and how I felt physically within my own body.

God set me free that day from the scale and its voice, and since then my health and my figure have continued to improve through making healthy choices and keeping an active lifestyle outside of what the scale has to say. So keep your heart open, because God loves you enough to pull you into the healthiest place you can be physically, emotionally and spiritually, if you will stay open to taking the deeper journey with Him.

The victorious heart

20 Others, like seed sown on good soil, hear the word, accept it, and produce a crop — some thirty, some sixty, some a hundred times what was sown.

R = RUN TO GOD

In the last part of the parable of the sower, we find out about those who were victorious, who cleared the hurdles of doubt, disappointment and distraction, and stepped into all that God had for them. The key statements in the scripture when translated from the original Greek language they were written in are that they, "heard the word" , meaning "take heed", and they "accepted it," which is the Greek word , which translates as "made it their own."

So they took heed of what was spoken to them and they made it their own, and it produced a crop of increase in their lives. Truly, this is the journey of encounter that we have explored in this book.

So in closing, I would like to summarize the EWL core values from the perspective of someone who is walking in victory and has completed the journey and brought forth a harvest, such as is described in this parable.

E = Eat Real Food / N = Nutrition Matters

They have learned to encounter food the right way, honoring their bodies and health, removing excess sugar and man-made, chemically laden concoctions from their diet. They are now feeding their bodies real food, increasing their health, wellbeing and longevity through strategic nutrition because it matters.

C = Connect With Others

They have come to recognize the patterns of isolation and withdrawal that can hold them back from freedom. So they are faithfully connected to others, walking in accountability and cheering on others towards success, having learned that encountering others is an essential a part of their journey.

O = Open Up

They have learned to open up to other people, to God and to new experiences and foods. They have taken off their masks, taken back their voices, and are courageously speaking the truth about what is happening in their journey. Their hearts are open and soft before the Lord and full of faith, hope and joy spilling the fruit of the spirit onto others.

U = *Understand Yourself*

They have come to understand themselves, having bravely confronted the layers involved in emotional eating and have learned skills and strategies to deal with the temptations, stressors and relationship issues in their lives. They have taken the deeper journey to deal with the past, learning to forgive and release the pain under the surface that has been a trigger for emotional eating. And in doing this, they have come into encounter with their real, authentic, God-given, beautiful self.

N = *No Guilt, No Shame, No Perfectionism*

They have broken free from the cycle of guilt, shame and perfectionism that had kept them trapped in yo-yo dieting, trapped by number on the scale, and trapped in a cycle of *"try hard and give up"*. They have stepped into God's grace, learning to be forgiving and gentle with themselves and to believe that God will give them His strength and power for the completion of this journey.

T = *Take Back Your Dreams*

They have taken back the dreams that had been lost along the way and moved from being spectators in life to participants. They have found a more powerful reason than the number on the scale to get to their goal, by identifying the things that God has called them to do in helping others and making a difference in the world. They are now pursuing health as a necessary part of having the energy and strength to complete God's Kingdom assignments.

E = *Exercise As A Lifestyle*

They have made exercise a lifestyle, neither ignoring it completely or turning it into an obsession. It has found its rightful place as an expression of joyful connection with life and a path to ongoing mobility and longevity.

R = *Run To God*

They have cleared the hurdles of doubt, disappointment and distraction and have learned to run to God whenever one of these obstacles come their way. They have taken the journey with Him, letting God into every part of their lives and hearts, so that at the end of the journey, they have found themselves in a place of abounding joy and fruitfulness, now enjoying the harvest of taking the deeper journey with Him.

They Have Encountered God

They Have Encountered Each Other

They Have Encountered Health and Nutrition

They Have Encountered Themselves,

and so…

They Have Encountered Weight Loss

RUN TO GOD — MY STORY

I started this book by talking about the difference between quick-fix and permanent change, which in reality is the difference between a powerless mindset verses a powerful one.

In looking back at my own life, I can see that when I started my weight-loss journey, I had all of the characteristics of a powerless mindset. I felt defeated on the inside and continually believed the answer was out there somewhere, rather than within myself. I bought into the lie that if only I could find the right diet or supplement I would be thin. This powerless mindset and belief system about weight loss ruled my thinking for years, and without God's intervention, I would likely have continued in it for the rest of my life.

But God, in His love and mercy, called me into the deeper journey, and so leaving those old defeating patterns behind I stepped out into new territory. I courageously allowed Him to peel back the layers of my soul and reveal the mindsets of doubt, discouragement and distraction that had sabotaged me over and over in my attempts to lose weight. I was stepping into a whole new way of dealing with a problem that had defeated me all of my life. It wasn't always easy, but it was authentic and real and the change has been permanent.

I have learned to allow God to deal with my heart, and teach me not only how to deal with daily stress, but also to face up to the deeper questions in life that so many of us avoid along the way.

I have learned to identify what I really want out of life, and have the courage to bring about necessary endings to those roles and relationships that were not fruitful for me. I have learned to take back my dreams and lay hold of a more powerful reason than the number on the scale to lose weight.

These have been real keys to breakthrough along the way. And by facing up to *the beasts in the basement,* those deep wounds I had been carrying for years that would trigger me to emotionally eat seemingly out of nowhere, I have felt a transformative experience that has brought me great freedom and peace.

To the best of my ability I have taken the deeper journey. With nutrition, with myself, with others and most importantly with God, and the results speak for themselves. I am free of food addiction, joyful in my soul and consistently at a healthy body weight that I now find easy to maintain. If you would have told me years back when I was utterly trapped by food, emotional pain and hopelessness that this day would come, I would have had a very hard time believing it was possible.

Yet each week as I look out at the faces of the many people that this

R = RUN TO GOD

program has helped to find their way to freedom, I am reminded once again that God can take the most broken places in our lives and make them into something beautiful and worthwhile.

So that's the end of my weight-loss story, and hopefully the beginning of yours. It is my desire that the Encounter Weight Loss program, both through this book, and through our online resourses, will be the fuel that will help you to take the deeper journey and encounter your weight loss too!

ACKNOWLEDGMENTS

I would like to thank all of those who helped me in the journey along the way to the completion of this project.

First and foremost Murray Peter my husband and biggest fan who has cheered me on every step of the way during this project and my kids who help me to find my "why" on the journey and continue to encourage me to use my voice as an influencer.

Kathy Sanderson who acted as my faithful assistant in the development phase of Encounter Weight Loss and provided honest and helpful feedback about what was working and what needed changing in the program.

To Micheal McIntee who poured hundreds of hours into images, charts, layouts and everything else that needs to be completed from a graphics point of view in a project like this.

To Susan, Brenda, Jennifer and others who edited and re-edited and told me what did not make sense.

To Helen who has always been there as a wonderful and wise encourager.

To every student who has taken the Encounter Weight Loss program and found freedom, thank you for the honor of serving you and being a part of your journey. It is a joy to see you step into freedom and that is my "why" for this project.

OTHER RESOURCES BY WENDY PETER

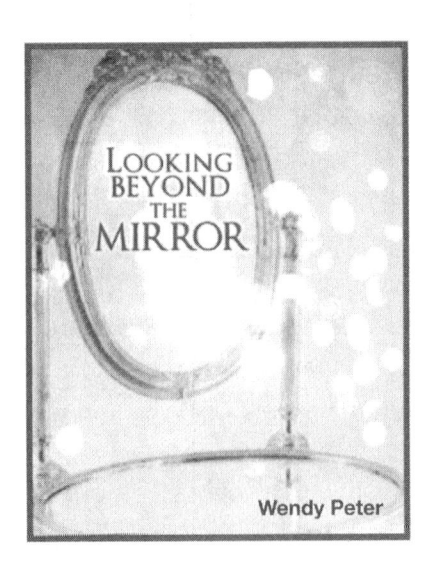

LOOKING BEYOND THE MIRROR

Too many women have received teaching on identity over the years and still have issues and yet still struggle with self-esteem issues. Its time for that to change. This in-depth audio course and workbook, will examine the ways our identities develop from the ground up.

You will learn how to confront and challenge any distorted messages you have picked up throughout your life journey. This transformational course will help you move beyond those distorted messages and the many expectations placed on you by others. Helping you come to rest in God's love and take hold of a lasting sense of confidence and self-esteem.

Available at www.wendypeter.com

ABOUT THE AUTHOR

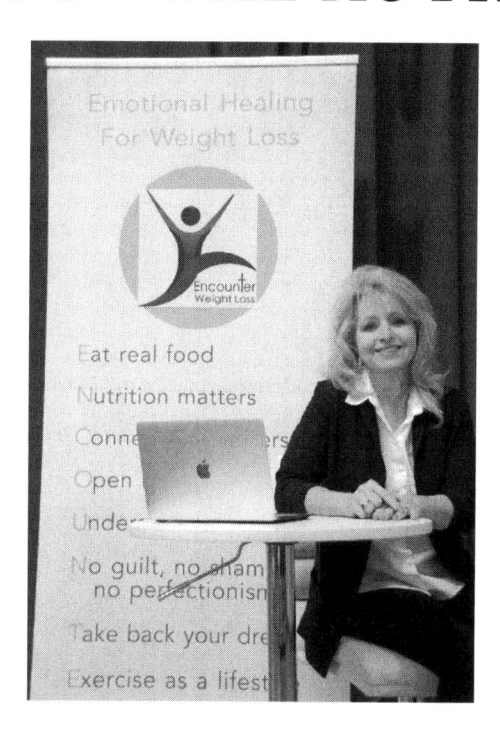

Wendy Peter is the North American Director of Women on the Frontlines and a Pastor at The Wave church in Winnipeg Manitoba.

She is an inspiring communicator, life coach and, teacher. She has spent her life empowering others to break free from the limitations and beliefs that have heard them back.

She is passionate above all about living from a place of intimacy with God and authenticity with others.

She is building Women on the Frontlines into a global movement that empowers, equips and mobilizes women into their destinies so that they can make a difference.

Wendy has been married to Murray for 35 years and they have three adult children.

ABOUT THE DESIGNER

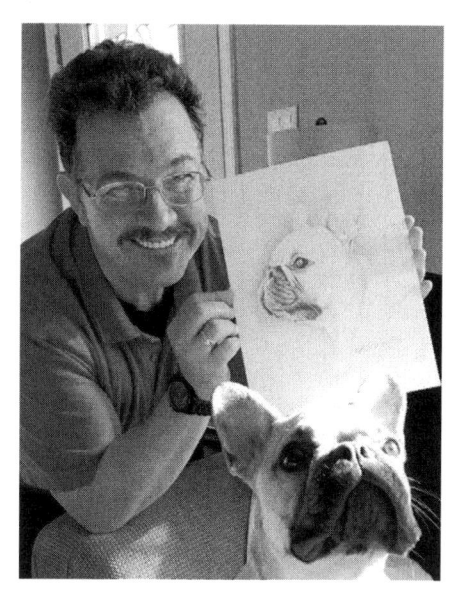

Michael P. McIntee is a talented freelance pencil illustrator and graphic designer.

He has been drawing for most of his life. His mother said that, "Michael started drawing when he discovered what a crayon and a wall could do together."

Born and raised in Ontario, Canada, he migrated to Saskatchewan in 2006 and now resides in rural Manitoba.

Aside from drawing, Michael enjoys teaching the fundamentals of art and spending quality time with his family.

Visit www.mypencilart.ca for more of Michael's work.

ENCOUNTERWEIGHTLOSS.COM